# THE GUINEA PIG CLUB

was formed on July 20th, 1941, at the Queen Victoria Hospital, East Grinstead. Its members were:

1. The Guinea Pigs (patients – fliers who, mutilated by burns, suffered and hoped in Sir Archibald McIndoe's Maxilio-Facial Unit).
2. The Scientists (doctors, surgeons and members of the medical staff).
3. The Royal Society for Prevention of Cruelty to Guinea Pigs (those friends and benefactors who by their interest in the hospital and patients make the life of the Guinea Pig a happy one).

Thirty-two years later the Guinea Pig Club is still in existence, and its story is an exciting and inspiring one – a story of courage and endurance, told here with vigour and understanding.

# The Guinea Pig Club

Edward Bishop

**NEW ENGLISH LIBRARY**
TIMES MIRROR

First published by Macmillan & Co. Ltd., in Great Britain 1963
© Edward Bishop 1963

*

FIRST NEL PAPERBACK EDITION AUGUST 1973
Reprinted, December 1973

*

*NEL Books are published by*
*New English Library Limited from Barnard's Inn, Holborn, London, E.C.1.*
*Made and printed in Great Britain by Hunt Barnard Printing Ltd., Aylesbury, Bucks.*

45001544 0

# ACKNOWLEDGEMENTS

This story contains some very personal information. For the fact that I have been privileged to present such information I am indebted to the committee of the Guinea Pig Club, to members of the club collectively, to many individual Guinea Pigs and, in particular, to the Chief Guinea Pig.

Much of the information was volunteered verbally, or was written information from members of the Guinea Pig Club, or appeared in *Guinea Pig*, the club magazine. But some of the information has come from the correspondence of the Guinea Pig Club and I wish, especially, to record my indebtedness to the committee for offering access to such information.

Some members, alas, have died since July 1941, and others cannot be traced. But the committee, in the true spirit of 'guinea-piggery', made available to me information about all members, so that a representative story could be told.

I thank, also, Lady McIndoe and Air Vice-Marshal Sir John Cordingley, formerly Controller of the Royal Air Force Benevolent Fund, for their encouragement and advice. This book was first published in 1963.

E.B.

The quotations at the beginning of
each chapter (excepting Chapter Eight) are taken from
the speeches and writings of the
late Sir Archibald McIndoe.

# CONTENTS

# FOREWORD

## by the late

SIR ARCHIBALD H. McINDOE
In a message to the magazine *Guinea Pig*, April, 1948.

One day someone will tell the complete story of Ward III* in the way it should be told.

Richard Hillary, Tom Gleave and Bill Simpson have told their personal experiences, but there is a wider field than the purely personal one. The future writer will tell of the return of the men of Dunkirk, tired but undismayed, who found their first rest there; of the Battle of Britain fought overhead, and the burned pilots who came to regard the place as home, gave it its particular flavour and then went back to fight carrying a card inscribed 'In case of further trouble deliver the bits to Ward III, East Grinstead . . .'.

Throughout the ups and downs of the war . . . Ward III sat more or less in the front line, a hive of activity, always busy, never dull.

He will tell of the Guinea Pig Club, how and why it started, what it achieved and what has become of all the Guinea Pigs who did not go down to defeat but rose from defeat to victory. Perhaps too, of the vast gifts which came from America, Canada, Australia, South Africa and New Zealand, and recognise the sacrifice of those who went back to fight and who encountered The Last Enemy. . . .

Had there been no Ward III there would not be today the great hospital which is making a real contribution to international understanding and friendship. . . .

This is the story to be told before the name that was Ward III sinks into oblivion. It is a great story and worthy of the telling.

*The birthplace of the Guinea Pig Club.

# PROLOGUE

Some wear dinner-jackets. Some wear suits. Some look prosperous and are. Some look prosperous and are not. None look as badly off as some are. But an odd-man-out at their Dinner, a whole, unscathed man, will recall such appearances later.

Here at table, one of the long finger tables leading from the knuckle table where sit the Chief Guinea Pig, the Controller of the R.A.F. Benevolent Fund, the chief philanthropists, the chief surgeons, the chief physicians, it is the sight of the hands which mesmerises the uninitiated. Stumps, knuckles, contracted claws. Hands that have been roasted. Raw, red and tissued. They are not paraded with the cringing ostentation of crippled beggars, but rest placidly, confidently at table, the old wounds the more savage for the whiteness of the tablecloths.

The odd man, the whole man bearing the legs, arms, hands, fingers, eyes and hair, nose and ears with which he was born, shifts his legs gingerly in the knowledge that under the table there are injured feet in heavy surgical boots, and government legs which are taken off every night, complete with shoes and socks.

Then, carrying enough Dutch courage to meet his hosts eye to eye (or eye to glass or plastic eye) the guest at the annual dinner of the Guinea Pig Club learns that talk releases a personality from behind each mask of facial plastic surgery. Meeting the men within he forgets the scars, the flaccid grafted skin, the wigs, the immobile masks which here and there bizarrely resemble the painted expression of a circus clown. He remembers that the outward appearance of the men at table may be the legacy of less than one minute in a burning, exploding, crashing war plane and of many years in and out of the Queen Victoria Hospital at East Grinstead.

This was one of the thoughts passing through this author's mind as he observed his hosts, the men who had asked him to write of their club, eating and drinking in the individual style to which each Guinea Pig had adapted those moving parts

11

which remained to him. Often it has returned – to be joined by these words:

> 'We do well to remember
> that the privilege of
> dying for one's country
> is not equal to the privilege
> of living for it.'

The valediction to his Guinea Pigs of the late Sir Archibald Hector McIndoe.

# CHAPTER ONE

'The development of this unique organisation from a meeting of the "Few" in 1941 round a bottle of sherry to its present flourishing condition is one of the curiosities of the war.'

Tom Gleave, who is the Chief Guinea Pig, asked, 'Will you write a book about the Guinea Pig Club? Not about Archie McIndoe. But the book *he* always wanted. The story of his Guinea Pigs. The men he re-made and who, as he often reminded people, helped to make him.'

Tom's face, hands, arms and legs were burned in the Battle of Britain: 'standard Hurricane burns' Tom calls them. A German cannon shell hit the fuel tank of his fighter in 1940.

Archie McIndoe gave Tom a new nose and there is a large patch of pale, dead-looking skin on Tom's forehead to show you where his nose came from. The patch looks dead because the skin which replaced the skin of Tom's new nose is foreign to those parts. It came from his thigh.

The new nose was the major job in Tom Gleave's facial repair. It is a large, healthy looking nose and because the skin of one's nose and of one's forehead is very much of the same texture it will redden obligingly after a pint or two of best bitter. Or of 'ordinary' for that matter. Tom's skin, like the rankless society of the Guinea Pig Club, accepts no distinctions.

Towards the end of 1940, Tom Gleave began his 'tour of ops' at the Queen Victoria Hospital, East Grinstead, but he was not then known as a member of 'McIndoe's Army', a Guinea Pig. The airmen began to call themselves Guinea Pigs that Christmas, but the club was not to be born until the following summer.

Surgically the growing of Tom's new nose is known as a rhinoplasty. Archie McIndoe curled the skin from the Squadron-Leader's forehead and grew it where the fire in the Hurricane cockpit had so consumed Tom's nose that it had shrivelled the nostrils into two tiny holes by his eyes.

Tom said, 'At the beginning of the war it was thought that

the best thing to do with badly injured airmen was to tuck them away quietly in a country institution where they would never be seen again and would be spared having to face the world. It seemed kinder to protect us from the public gaze and it was also believed that the sight of chaps like us would depress the public and with them the general war morale.'

Tom's half-moon spectacles slid to the tip of the nose that Archie McIndoe had grown and sculptured for him at East Grinstead more than twenty years earlier. The fire in his Hurricane had caught Tom's eyelashes and burned away the eyelids which had saved his eyes. Watering, friendly, tired eyes. Tired, perhaps, by the wartime Whitehall papers which Tom reads as an official war historian. Like the majority of the survivors of 'McIndoe's Army', Tom is – as he says – 'up to his new eyelids in work'. He is not tucked away in an institution. East Grinstead and the Guinea Pig Club changed all that.

\* \* \*

The Guinea Pig Club was born of the Sunday morning hangover which most of Ward III at the East Grinstead hospital had earned on the night of July 19th, 1941. 'Let's have a grogging party' somebody said. Those who could move, shuffled to a hut next door where the surgeons kept a 'mess', and a Czech fighter pilot, Frankie Truhlar, uncorked a bottle of sherry. There would have been other willing barmen had there been hands but Frankie Truhlar was the only patient in a sufficiently advanced state of repair to play host.

The clouds above East Grinstead parted to unration the sun, but for the men from Ward III the sherry was more warming than the sun. Ward III was not a large airy ward like the picture-windowed wards along the front of this modern cottage hospital. The most mutilated airmen of the war were in a little brown wooden army hut, at the back of the main hospital buildings.

It is popularly believed that the late Sir Archibald McIndoe, 'the Boss' or 'the Maestro' as his Guinea Pigs knew him, brilliantly conceived the idea of the Guinea Pig Club. This was not so. When the sherry had submerged the hangovers on that Sunday morning in 1941 the heavily bandaged fliers decided that, as they enjoyed their own company at these grogging parties, they would form a 'grogging club'. In hospital nomenclature McIndoe's operating theatre and the little wooden hut comprised a Maxilio-Facial

14

Unit. Correspondingly, the minutes of the Grogging Club were headed, 'The Maxillonian Club whose members call themselves Guinea Pigs'.

Pilot-Officer Geoffrey Page, subsequently he was to return to the hospital as a Squadron-Leader with fresh wounds, had been 'fried' over the channel during the Battle of Britain. He recorded the minutes of the meeting.

'The objects of the Club are to promote good fellowship among, and to maintain contact with, approved frequenters of Queen Victoria Cottage Hospital.

'There are three classes of membership, all having equal rights:
1. The Guinea Pigs (patients).
2. The Scientists (doctors, surgeons and members of the medical staff).
3. The Royal Society for Prevention of Cruelty to Guinea Pigs. (Those friends and benefactors who by their interest in the hospital and patients make the life of the Guinea Pig a happy one.)

'The annual subscription for all members is 2/6, due on the 1st July each year. Women are not eligible for membership, but a 'ladies' evening may be held at the direction of the Committee.

'The following members were proposed and seconded by members present.

President: Mr A. H. McIndoe, F.R.C.S.

Vice-President: Squadron Leader T. Gleave.

Secretary: F/O. W. Towers Perkins.

Treasurer: P/O. P. C. Weeks.

Committee members: Messrs. Coote, Edmonds, Page, Hughes, Wilton, Overeyander, Gardiner, Russell Davies, Fraser, Hunter, Eckoff, Morley and Livingstone.

'Other members present were: Messrs McLeod, Mappin, Clarkson and Bodenham.

'The following were proposed and seconded as members: Messrs Dewar, Shephard, Lock, Hillary, Fleming, Lord, Hart, Langdale, Bennions, Harrison, Butcher, Truhlar, Kokal, Noble, Mann, Krasnordebski, McPhail, Banham and Smith-Barry.'

At the time none of the men in the black iron beds in the brown wooden hut were aware of the movement they had started. Nor could McIndoe or Gleave have imagined the serious burden those titles of President and Vice-President, light-hearted as they appeared in the context of a 'Grogging Club', were to lay upon them for the rest of their lives. Nor, certainly that after the

15

death of Archie McIndoe their new 'Boss' would be a young prince serving at sea in the Royal Navy, as junior in the Service and as unknown as themselves.

That the principal purpose of the club at this point was to give a little more meaning to the East Grinstead grogging sessions is shown by the reasons advanced at the time for the respective appointments of Bill Towers Perkins and Peter Weeks. The secretary was picked because, physically, he could not write and the treasurer because, being unable to walk, he could not make off with the funds.

In the glow of the sherry the Maxillonians showed perception. Twenty-one years afterwards the Guinea Pig Club is proud of what it has achieved with a minimum of paper work. Until ten years ago it had raised and lent £11,000, a process which was much aided by those Guinea Pigs who had made repayments of £7,500 and thus, by keeping the money moving round and round, had themselves provided help for fellow Pigs. In addition, it had donated as grants, nearly £11,000. It had also introduced about £250,000 to its greatest benefactor, the R.A.F. Benevolent Fund, from which its members had benefited to the extent of more than £60,000 in grants and loans. Since that time, as its members grew older, the Club's achievements have expanded.

\* \* \*

There must have been many wartime drinking sessions among the Services at which the most solemn of pledges were taken to meet regularly and to remain a band of brothers. A club. Some of these Service 'grogging clubs' died with the next day's hangover. Others lingered and disappeared with the last shillings of the gratuity. Few survived.

It is doubtful if the Guinea Pigs could have been born in hospital conditions other than those which the early Pigs, encouraged by McIndoe, helped to create for themselves at East Grinstead. One says 'encouraged by McIndoe' because grogging clubs are not regarded as normal routine in hospitals, civil or Service.

Ward III itself was peculiarly conducive to the development of a club atmosphere. To the unwelcome, but traded upon, rarity of being a very badly burned airman, the ward added the exclusivity of being just a little wooden hut. As a gang of smugglers might have remembered their deepest cave, so in their

16

own way the Guinea Pigs draw inspiration from the hut which became a 'sty'.

The creation of this spirit was helped also by the ward's reception of men wounded in two of the most stirring episodes of British history, Dunkirk and the Battle of Britain. Years afterwards, when Guinea Pigs had burst the plank walls of Ward III and spread into the new and more conventional (only in the architectural sense) wards which the Canadians and Americans were to add to the hospital at East Grinstead, Archie McIndoe would cite specific Pigs as *his* reason for starting the Guinea Pig Club. He never intended to steal the credit for the club but he never passed up an opportunity, with a little white lying if necessary, to present a very badly injured Pig as his reason for the club, if he thought this would strengthen the airman's case for a higher disability pension or a particular job.

Let it be recognised, therefore, that as the surgeon has written, 'The development of this unique organisation from a meeting of the "Few" in 1941 round a bottle of sherry . . . is one of the curiosities of the war'.

The Guinea Pig Club was as brilliantly unplanned as any of Britain's best success stories! Certainly no official mind could have decreed:

'We'll put the burned airmen in an uncomfortable wooden hut at the back of the Queen Victoria Cottage Hospital. There they will create an amazing spirit, bringing to it the spirit of the fighter squadrons.

'Then, when we get more and more burned airmen from the heavy bombers – among some of whom the morale may not be so high because they will not be the cream like these chaps – the spirit will have wafted through the hospital and everybody will get better much quicker as a result of our ingenious plan. Gracious heavens, some may even return to the war and use again the killing skills which it has cost the nation so much time and money to teach them.

'Meanwhile, just to help the chaps along we'll recruit the prettiest nurses we can find for this very special hospital and we'll put a fellow called McIndoe in charge of the lot because he seems not only pretty capable at carving people up but also to understand their minds – and it is every bit as important to understand people as to graft their skin when dealing with burns cases.

'Oh yes, one more very important point. We should find a

hospital where the Matron will be a thoroughly good sort, smile sweetly and take Mr McIndoe in her stride. She must welcome beer-barrels in the wards and will not have to mind when some of her patients return from the London night-clubs in time for breakfast.

'The cottage hospital of East Grinstead then, is entirely suitable. Matron Hall is a poppet and has a talent for turning a blind eye.

'Ah, another point. Anaesthesia for plastic surgery is a specialised branch of medicine and like Mr McIndoe the anaethetists must be humanitarians. Team up Dr John Hunter and Dr Russell Davies.

'Finally, East Grinstead is a good healthy spot. Fresh clean Sussex air. Not too far from the night spots of London so that we can keep the chaps cheered up. There are also the scented pinewoods around. Mr McIndoe says they contain healing properties, better still for Guinea Pigs, they enclose the homes of some of the wealthiest inhabitants of Great Britain. McIndoe enjoys the social life and he's just the man to persuade the rich to do the chaps well once they're on their crutches. A club? That's a top priority!'

Such perception would have been to much to expect of the official British mind.

It has been a grinding labour to separate truth from legend in seeking out the story of the Guinea Pig Club (and one cannot promise that one has always managed to do so) but the club says, and one defers to its belief, that under the government's Emergency Medical Services scheme the Maxilio-Facial Unit came to 'E.G.' because the responsible surgeon – not the late Sir Archibald McIndoe – found the Queen Victoria Hospital geographically convenient for visits to his son at a nearby preparatory school.

* * *

'Throughout the ups and downs of the war . . . Ward III sat more or less in the front line . . .' the Boss reminded Guinea Pigs in his message to the first number of their magazine. The hospital at Orpington to which Tom Gleave's 'fried' body was delivered after he had defended London was even more in the front line than East Grinstead during the Battle of Britain.

Tom had been leading an attack on a formation of Ju 88

bombers when his Hurricane caught fire. He reported, 'A long spout of flame was issuing from the hollow starboard wing-root, curling up along the port side of the cockpit and then across towards my right shoulder. I had some crazy notion that if I rocked the aircraft and skidded, losing speed, the fire might go out. Not a bit of it. The flames increased until the cockpit was like the centre of a blow-lamp nozzle. There was nothing left to do but bale out. A forced landing was out of the question as I was still 7,000 to 8,000 feet up. I reached down to pull the radio telephone lead out of its socket but the heat was too great. The skin was already rising off my right wrist and hand and my left hand was starting to blister, the glove being already partially burnt off. My shoes and slacks must have been burning all this time but I cannot remember any great pain.'

Squadron-Leader Gleave undid his cockpit harness and tried to raise himself. Finding he was too weak he was prepared to shoot himself if he could not escape. He flew with a loaded revolver. He pulled off his helmet, though this was not without a struggle and opened the cockpit cover. He had decided to roll the Hurricane on to her back and to hope to fall out but before he could complete the manoeuvre there was a great flash and his burning body was thrown clear, almost as if one of the modern ejector seats had been heard of in 1940. It seemed to Tom that he was travelling through yards of flame, turning over and over in the air but with no sense of falling. He found the rip-cord handle and it was only later that he realised that the fire and his escape had happened in less than a minute. A pilot did not survive more than a minute in a blazing Hurricane.

\*　　\*　　\*

When the sirens sounded patients at Orpington were placed under their beds. The first time Tom 'came-to' after an emergency operation, he found himself under a bed. 'There's a battle going on overhead', said 'Blossom' his nurse.

That night his night nurse told him, 'We have several R.A.F. pilots in the hospital as well as many Dunkirk casualties'. The siren sounded again as she was speaking and Tom was lifted out of bed and back into his private 'shelter'. The floor shook as the anti-aircraft guns opened up and Tom could hear the whistle of bombs. His nurse knelt beside him. When the bombs were falling she put one hand on his shoulder and the other on the

19

cage over his burned legs, sprawling herself protectingly across him.

Tom remembers, 'There was a terrific crump. Then another and another. The building seemed repeatedly to leave the ground and come back, thud, thud, thud.

'Then came a lull. I asked for a drink and some ice. My mouth was parched and the corners of it seemed to tear apart as I tried to speak. Nurse brought a bowl of ice cubes and a glass of iced water. Then she placed some ice in my mouth, repeating this every ten minutes. It was delicious.

'Again we heard the drone of the Hun and then the bombs came crashing down around us. It went on for hours and all the time my nurse crouched beside me, placing more ice in my mouth and adjusting my pillow from time to time.'

Then she gave Tom a sleeping draught. Such a badly injured man could have too much of the 'front line'.

Tom Gleave continues his story:

'One afternoon – it may have been the next day – I was awake. Sister said that my wife had arrived.

'I was well enough to worry about Beryl seeing me as I was. My hands, forehead and legs were encased in dried tannic acid. My face, which felt the size of the proverbial melon, was treated in the same way and I peered through slits in the mask.

'I heard footsteps approaching the bed and then saw my wife standing gazing at me. She flushed a little and said, "What on earth have you been doing with yourself, darling?" "Had a row with a German", I replied.

'She tried to smile and sat down by my side. It was not until I saw my face in a mirror weeks later that I realised how brave she had been.'

Like many of his fellow 'fried' Pigs, Tom Gleave, the Chief Guinea Pig, passed several weeks in a delirium. 'A world, half real, half fanciful', he says. 'I can remember some times when "Blossom" would bend over me and I would find something different about her. For it would be Beryl.'

One night when the nurses had lowered Tom into his air-raid shelter, he thought he was in a room where the ceiling was very low and people were walking about ducking their heads. 'I became involved in a heated argument and a fight, people were trying to hold me down but I lashed out, sometimes burying my hands in the ceiling and bringing plaster down on the floor.'

Emerging from the delirium, Tom found his night nurse exhausted and that the tannic acid on his hands had flaked away in his battle with her and the bed-springs overhead.

Tom's delirious period was ending when he was told that a new treatment for burns which did not involve tannic acid, was being given at a special unit at East Grinstead and he was to be transferred to that hospital because it specialised also in skin grafting and plastic surgery.

When Archie McIndoe examined Tom's face at East Grinstead he told him, 'We can do either of two things with that nose of yours. We can graft a piece of skin on to it and give it some sort of covering. Or, we can give you a new nose. This latter method will be quite a big job but well worth it.' Tom took the new nose.

It was not until his first leave from the hospital that Tom became conscious of the effect of his disfigured appearance upon other people and even then, feeling very much the same man inside, it seemed to him at first that they were staring at 'a fellow wearing a great-coat that was now two or three sizes too big for him and a collar that showed a wide gap all round'. He was helped, he says, by the Maestro's observation, 'They can get used to it and *like* it!'

In the middle of repair Tom was told that he looked a more terrifying sight than he would when all his plastic surgery had been completed and he confronted himself by thinking, 'Go on, have a good look. I won't be like this much longer.'

In any event, there was another matter which was worrying him very much more than the horror or compassion of strangers in the street.

A regular officer and commander of a fighter squadron, he had temporarily lost his sense of self respect, a loss which owed nothing to his disfigurement. 'It rankled to have been shot down', he remembers. 'I was touchy about being out of the war, which was not conducive to an even temper – but Beryl took it all in her stride. Only once did I come near to lifting the lid off the pot. I was doing some short-range shopping for Beryl which took me to a little bread shop. I shuffled in and asked for a loaf. The lady behind the counter took one look at my face and quickly forgot my order. "And what have you been doing sonny?" she asked. "I had a spot of bother up there", I said, pointing upwards. "Oh well", she said, "I suppose you did your best".'

* * *

Some of the names which were among those in the minutes of

the 'Grogging Club' will have been recognised, notably that of Richard Hillary, whose book 'The Last Enemy' in which he tells of Ward III, is already a classic of war literature. But only those whose memories return to the first war and who can recognise the distinguished tie of the Royal Flying Corps, or who can recall the Gosport system of flying instruction will remember the double-barrelled name of its protagonist which appeared at the end of the list: Smith-Barry.

All those on the list – the burned airmen, the 'scientists', the members of 'The Royal Society for the Prevention of Cruelty to Guinea Pigs' – all had good reason to be on the list. All, with the exception of the veteran Royal Flying Corps pilot, Robert Smith-Barry. A patient who should never have been at the hospital, Smith-Barry, inadvertently was greatly to influence the future and serious mission of the Guinea Pig Club.

McIndoe had been very doubtful about the propriety of sparing a bed for Smith-Barry, although had he known the future benefit a developing friendship with this resourceful, veteran airman was to bring the club, he would – with his usual opportunism – have assured Smith-Barry not only of a bed but of a red carpet all the way there from the ambulance. As it was, the surgeon felt that he had been bounced into receiving this patient.

McIndoe had answered the telephone to the wealthy Colonel Phillipi, a Flying Corps friend of Smith-Barry's in the first war.

'Mr McIndoe? Good. Now look here, I want you to provide a private room, a beautiful nurse, a vi-sprung mattress and your personal attention four times a day for a friend called Smith-Barry. He's already been in two hospitals and he had himself removed because he doesn't like being messed about. Now he wants to come to East Grinstead.'

Smith-Barry had heard of Ward III's reputation as a remarkable haven where hospitalised individuals could remain individuals and he was the first of a number of airmen who were to 'organise' – in the wartime meaning of that word – an escape from the rigours of ordinary hospitals and achieve admittance at the Queen Victoria Cottage Hospital – The Sty.

In later years, it amused Archie McIndoe, employing his effulgent, after-a-good-dinner technique, to recall the manner of Smith-Barry's arrival. 'If I remember', he would say, 'I was fairly hostile to the whole idea and even more so when a spanking great ambulance arrived complete with two obvious old hands from World War I, of whom I had never heard.

'Such, however, was the charm of manner of George Phillipi that my irritation was rapidly allayed, the private room and nurse were produced, the soft bed supplied and I found myself visiting Robert Smith-Barry more than four times a day.

'One day Smith-Barry came to me and said that his ancient carcass could be of little use to the Air Force and could I and would I, use it as a source of skin for the young men under my care. As gently as possible I told him there was only one Smith-Barry and that his skin was no use but that if he really wanted to help me, he could come to East Grinstead and act as a sort of liaison officer between Air Ministry and E.G. Promptly he said that in the field of negotiation he was no good at all but that his friend George Phillipi was superb at it and he would persuade him to come.'

The Guinea Pig Club, in embryo, persuaded the Air Force of the need for an office at the Air Ministry to care for its welfare problems and very soon a department, invented by the Guinea Pig Club and intriguingly named P.5., appeared at Adastral House. To run it, Colonel George Phillipi, freshly commissioned as an unusually venerable Pilot-Officer.

With Pilot-Officer Phillipi looking after the Pigs' interests at Ministry and elsewhere, it was necessary for him to talk day-to-day detail with somebody other than Mr McIndoe at East Grinstead. He found 'Blackie'.

# CHAPTER TWO

'Blackie was a natural in the field of human relationship and is today, in my opinion, one of the really great experts in the business.'

'Blackie' is not the name of a dog Guinea Pig. It is the Guinea Pigs' name for Edward Blacksell, for many years Headmaster of the Barnstaple Secondary Modern School, a director of the English Stage Company (The Royal Court Theatre) and the large, shaggy dogsbody to the Guinea Pig Club, which he became 32 years ago when he arrived at Ward III with his P.T. kit.

Smith-Barrie's gallant, if impractical, offer of his own skin, had brought Phillipi into guinea-piggery and Phillipi had sent for the man who could persuade young airmen to believe in P.T. – and anybody who once upon a time volunteered at less than twenty to fight the Germans will remember how time-wasting P.T. seemed to young men tearing their hearts out to win their wings and get into the war.

Thus a baffled 'Blackie', an assistant school-teacher from North Devon, who had done no serious P.T. before joining the R.A.F., found himself posted to the Queen Victoria Hospital, East Grinstead.

Blackie had hoped to join the Navy and it was only when the doctors rejected him that he volunteered for the R.A.F. and was recommended for training in that muscular world of ropes, weights and wall bars, the School for Physical Training Instructors.

His selection for this course came about in a curious fashion, although it will not appear odd to those Pigs who know how fate habitually tilts this lively man at life.

Blackie had reported at the former airship base of Cardington. There, standing tall, thin and with that anxious, slightly stooping, angle of attention of most tall recruits, he was interviewed by the type of resurrected officer one used to know as a 'Dug Out'.

The Dug Out, considering an R.A.F. 'trade' for the young school-teacher, who was in his early twenties, gazed out of the

24

window and at that moment saw a party of men marching some half a mile away. He beckoned Blackie outside. 'Shout at those men', he commanded. 'If you can persuade them to double over here, I've got a job for you'.

If there was one attribute which might serve Blackie well in the Air Force, it was his ability to make himself heard – and obeyed. When your schooldays are spent playing football at Barnstaple on a winter's day your lungs do battle with the wind from Exmoor. Those airmen, assuring Blackie's future as a Physical Training Instructor and unbeknown to them, the future of the Guinea Pig Club, doubled over.

Later came a posting to Plymouth to subdue some high-spirited Australians of No. 10 R.A.A.F. Squadron. Edward Blacksell rigged, as the Australians said, 'a bastard of an assault course', promising a barrel of beer which was to be consumed only when each and every man had beaten Blackie's time to complete it.

The challenge appealed to the Australians. When they had been tamed and the barrel drained dry, Sergeant Blacksell, to his astonishment, was ordered to report to Mr Archibald McIndoe at the Queen Victoria Hospital, East Grinstead.

'Good God', exclaimed a legless and horrified Guinea Pig when Blackie laid out his gym shoes, shorts and P.T. vest on a bed in Ward III, 'you're not something well doing P.T. with us!'

The pigs to their delight very soon discovered that the Sergeant was no knees-bend, arms-upward-stretch automaton. He enjoyed beer and it was obvious to them from the beginning that he was going to enjoy the hostilities which already had opened between them and the service authorities from beneath the McIndoe civilian umbrella.

One of the first battles took place shortly after Blackie's arrival. It is remembered by Pigs as 'The Battle of the Blues' because it was caused by the issue of, and the order to wear, government hospital blue uniforms and red ties.

The airmen were proud of their Air Force uniforms and the flying brevets they had earned. They feared that converted by the blues into hospitalised men they might be mistaken for army privates or even some special class of convicted prisoners. Pig Henry Standen comments, 'We were glad to fight for the flag but not to parade East Grinstead in it.'

The Boss agreed with the Pigs that the hospital blues were as out of date as hospitals without barrels of beer in the wards, and as the official description 'invalid' which persuaded a patient that he was a permanent cripple.

The Pigs collected the hospital blue uniforms and burned them on a bonfire with a blessing from the surgeon coupled with the advice, 'For heaven's sake don't spoil the blackout'. McIndoe did not want his aircrew repair shop blown to hell by enemy airmen.

The bonfire may have escaped the notice of the Germans but the smoke, like the coiling smoke signals of Red Indians did not escape the watchful guardians of good order and discipline.

An Air Ministry officer with a posse of Air Force police descended upon the disfigured wrecks of burned airmen who hobbled about the hostelries of East Grinstead in R.A.F. uniforms or any clothing they could muster – other than the detested hospital blues.

The strutting arrival of the belted and gaitered policemen, with their high germanesque-peak caps, short haircuts and highly polished chins, caused vast amusement among the 'mutinous' men who had been so mutilated in His Majesty's service. But while laughing, they also blessed McIndoe's decision never to accept the service rank with which Whitehall had attempted to invest him. Remaining a civilian surgeon at a civilian hospital, he could repel such attacks. And he did, as Australian Pig, George Taylor, remembers, 'reflecting his usual craftiness by preventing the authorities from bringing their plans to fruition'.

Archie McIndoe discovered that there had been issued an Air Ministry authority for all ranks to dress in sports clothes when going to sport. He arranged, therefore, that tennis courts, squash courts and a swimming pool in the area of East Grinstead should be open to his patients.

The service police were stymied, confronted as they were by the spectacle of disfigured men, heavily bandaged men, men on crutches, in wheelchairs, men helping each other along like boys in a three-legged race – all 'on our way to tennis and squash and to swimming'. The policemen turned about and were not seen again.

In any event, apart from the depressing influence they bore on the Pigs' morale, the government's hospital blues were impractical for some of the badly hurt men. Stiff government flybuttons are difficult to manoeuvre. Old, well-worn grey flannels are much handier and Guinea Pig life was later considerably eased when the Canadians sent over a stock of zips.

There was also the important consideration of the maintenance of the Guinea Pigs' rankless society. The Air Ministry's enforcement of blues for men below Warrant Officer rank but freedom for those more senior, was regarded as an affront to the club attitude which had developed from McIndoe's initial insistence that a badly burned man was a badly burned man irrespective of whether he was an Air Marshal or an A.C.2.

McIndoe always conceded that less freedom and more discipline would have provided better therapy for some of the Pigs. These, however, he numbered at about two per cent of the total and he did not intend to allow the Air Ministry to make ninety-eight per cent of his patients suffer for such a small minority.

\*   \*   \*

If Blackie possesses any ties other than the tie of the Guinea Pig Club – with its distinctive R.A.F. colours and winged Guinea Pig motif – then they must be a dull, mildewing collection. Blackie without his Guinea Pig tie would seem as naked as Gus Fowler, the Guinea Pig who joined a nudist colony.

Few unscathed men are privileged to wear the tie and Blackie's tie was not entirely unearned by bed-hours and plastic surgery, although neither his P.T. classes with the East Grinstead nurses, the only P.T. the Pigs allowed him at the Sty, nor the occasion when he was debagged and 'beaten-up' by convalescent Pigs at Marchwood Park, was the cause.

It was a very serious motor accident seven years ago which introduced Blackie to lengthy hospital treatment and plastic surgery. The fact that this did not take place at East Grinstead still invokes a round of mirth and drinks, at the annual Guinea Pig dinner. As the Boss told Pigs shortly after the accident, 'Blackie is lucky to be alive. He had a very unpleasant car accident and almost bought it. He is now really one of you. He had quite a bit of plastic surgery and I must say, they've done a darned good job on him, even though he did go to a rival firm.'

The rival firm was the Oldstock Hospital at Salisbury. Blackie was wearing his club tie when an ambulance delivered him to the hospital. His Guinea Pig Status rendered him a medical celebrity and earned him almost a red carpet all the way from 'Casualty' to the ward.

Some knowledge of the East Grinstead tradition and the Ward III spirit had reached this hospital. Blackie recalls, 'The words

27

"E.G." and "Guinea Pig" produced a respectful handling of the injured parts, a sweeping away of regulations . . .'.

The Matron, making her first ward round after Blackie's admission, stopped at his bed and observed to Sister that something was missing.

'This man', Matron said, 'is a Guinea Pig. He needs a pint of beer!'

Not long after Blackie recovered from his own plastic surgery he began to help a Guinea Pig whose situation serves well to introduce a theme which runs through all the actions of the Guinea Pig Club – readiness to provide personal and repeated reassurance to the same members long, long after the end of their service life.

In 1942 at the start of his career as a Guinea Pig, Alan Morgan, a young industrial apprentice from Manchester, had lain for days at East Grinstead in a very shocked and dazed condition.

He was little aware of what was happening to him except that he knew that the nurses insisted upon keeping his hands immersed in buckets of ice. He could not appreciate that the doctors were trying to save his hands so that he could follow his trade, and Blackie remembers that Alan's sole contribution to any attempt at conversation was, 'This is a bloody place and they're all bloody mad in here'.

What nobody knew at the time was in what circumstances all the fingers of young Alan Morgan, a Flight Engineer, had been turned into the black sticks which had to be kept immersed in a pair of ice buckets.

His bomber was high over Leipzig when it was attacked heavily by flak and the enemy fire burst open a door in the side of the aircraft. Two of his fellow aircrew, attempting to close the door, had passed out through lack of oxygen. Alan pulled them back from the dangerous opening and plugged them in to the oxygen supply to bring them round. Then Alan lost consciousness and, as at that moment the bomber was attacked by fighters, no one could pull him away from the open door where he had fallen, his gloveless hands hanging out over Germany.

Unlike most of the others in the ward whom he thought were 'bloody mad', Alan was not fried but frost-bitten.

In the end the surgeons decided that there was no chance of saving Alan's fingers, that the charcoal sticks were for the 'chop' as Guinea Pigs say.

On the day his name was on the list for the operation, Alan

beseeched Blackie to stay with him in the theatre while they took his fingers off. Blackie not only watched the operation but he wheeled Alan into the theatre on the hospital trolley. When the young air-gunner surfaced from the anaesthetic, Blackie was at his bedside to explain not how much the Maestro had removed but that he had left part of the thumb on each hand and what a help this would be when Alan began to learn to use what remained of his hands. Then Blackie wrote, at Alan's dictation, to Ella, his girl in Manchester.

* * *

Possibly more difficult during wartime than reassuring the Pigs, were Blackie's interviews with some of their friends and relations. Not all were as sympathetic to Blackie's personality as Ella. There was the day Jimmy Wright's father, an official war correspondent newsreel cameraman, came to see his son who had been burned beyond recognition and blinded in both eyes when his Marauder photographic-reconnaissance bomber exploded.

Mr Wright, in his job, was accustomed to some very courteous attention from the highest ranking officers wherever he filmed the war. When he arrived at East Grinstead, he was already in a fairly aggressive mood because previously, the Army had informed him that his son had died in an army hospital in Italy, an error which Mr Wright traced to this explanation: a Warrant Officer had considered it administratively more simple that night to notify Jimmy's death in a comprehensive casualty signal, it seeming obvious that no man, so badly burned, could survive until morning. In consequence, Jimmy's father recalls that he was very, very upset by the levity with which Blackie, 'only a Warrant Officer', played with a squash racket while he talked and scrutinised him with such an air of authority that he might have been the Chief of the Air Staff himself!

It is probable that had Jimmy remained alone in the Army's hands the message regretting his death on active service would have been substantiated. His father saved his son's life. With the help of a friendly American general, Mr Wright flew to Jimmy's side and found that he was being massively drugged. His experience of morphia in the Royal Flying Corps in the first war and as a front-line cameraman in the second, told him that such doses would not only release Jimmy from pain, but kill him. There was a dramatic moment at the hospital when Mr Wright at Jimmy's bedside seized a syringe just as a nurse was about to plunge it into his son and dashed it on the floor.

Jimmy's father, employing his status as a war correspondent, used all the influence he could muster to move his son home until, with Jimmy bandaged from head to foot like a mummy and packed between two aero-engines inside a freighting Liberator aircraft, Mr Wright flew with his son to England. There were some frightening moments over the heavily defended port of Brest but an escort of Spitfires arrived to see the Liberator home, and Flying-Officer Wright arrived in some style. His father without knowing anything about the Guinea Pig Club or how piratically it could operate, had saved his son in the true spirit of the club, of which Jimmy was to become one of the most popular, if not THE most popular member. The airman the Army had said was dead.

\* \* \*

Jimmy talked about his R.A.F. and Guinea Pig career in his house near the Thames at Shepperton. He took the house to be close to the film business he had built, a remarkable achievement for a blind man.

There he has looked after himself since the manservant he had hired took advantage of his blindness and stole from the house. This happened when Jimmy was in France, where the Guinea Pig Club had arranged special surgery in a final attempt to obtain a slight restoration of sight in one eye. Jimmy returned home to two disappointments. His man's disloyalty and the end of hope.

Jimmy insisted on a mug of beer. 'You can't talk to a Guinea Pig without a pint.' He poured out the beer and were it not for the glassy nothingness of his sky-blue eyes which, seeing nothing, are about all that remains of Jimmy's face, one would have said, 'This man CAN see'.

Generally, when one meets a totally or partially disfigured Guinea Pig, one finds oneself seeking communication through the eyes of the man. The face will tell you little or nothing about the Pig's emotions. Plastic surgeons can graft pieces of skin from donor areas elsewhere in the body but they cannot replace the little muscles, the movement of which contribute to a smile to charm or on the darker side of human personality, to the sneer or even the leer, according to a man's mental attitudes, before the fire consumed the facial expressions which were their advertisement.

Jimmy Wright's sightless eyes convey nothing. But his mouth was cleverly contrived by the Maestro and there is just enough movement in it to provide the smile which introduces the quality in Jimmy Wright which Blackie, who has known him so many years, describes as 'saintly'. There is a photograph of Jimmy in his medical file which shows him happy and smiling when he joined the R.A.F. It is a picture of a good looking young man, very pleased at being 'snapped' for the first time in his new uniform. This photograph guided McIndoe and his fellow plastic surgeons through the sixty operations they performed on Jimmy and, with the help of what remained of Jimmy Wright, they contrived a smile just like the one in the picture, the smile which has brought Jimmy so many friends and which cements the film business (he runs his own production company) which his ability attracts. It is a smile which after a few moments of conversation, almost convinces one that he is not blind because in one's imagination one sees the eyes light up with interest as he visualises the television commercial he is making or even the war which shattered him.

So many years after the war it is forgotten how much acceptance as aircrew in the Air Force meant to young men like Jimmy Wright. One could tuck the white flash of aircrew into one's forage cap and walk out of one's caste environment, high, low or middle, into the honoured, privileged, glamorised company of men where the dream of the eventual flying brevet completely discounted the actuarial expectation of a short, if gay, life.

On his eighteenth birthday Jimmy Wright had volunteered for aircrew but he received a big disappointment when, after his medical, he was told his eyesight was not good enough. The disappointment was heightened because, his father having stayed in the Air Force for ten years after the first war, Jimmy had grown up in R.A.F. camps.

It has happened many times in war that a man who has failed to gain acceptance in an arm of the Services which demands supreme medical fitness, has found himself more dangerously engaged than he would have been had he been fuller of breath, quicker of limb or sharper of sight. Jimmy Wright decided that as he could not join the R.A.F. as a potential pilot he would take a civilian job until his call-up papers arrived. He joined the Technicolor film firm and it was experience there that was to lead to an R.A.F. photographic course and to commissioned service as an operational film cameraman – and anybody who has seen any of the low-level attack filming of the R.A.F.'s bomber aircraft will appreciate the hazards of that occupation.

Before a member of the R.A.F. Film Unit could join an operational squadron he was ordered to qualify in some respect as aircrew so that in an emergency he could leave his camera and fight. Thus Jimmy achieved his ambition to become aircrew and, qualifying as an air-gunner, sewed the single-wing with the letters 'A.G.' on to the tunic of his new Pilot-Officer's uniform.

Pilot-Officer Wright, air-gunner, reported to the Pinewood film studios where his part of the R.A.F. unit was situated and he remembers that it seemed strange to be walking about the studios and film sets. Sometimes he wondered whether he was real and if his smart new uniform had not been provided by the wardrobe department. As no 'other ranks' bothered to salute he took the charitable view that *they* were the film extras.

Jimmy filmed his first bombing operations over France and the Low Countries and was posted to the Desert Air Force where he found a cool welcome. He recalls, 'No. 223 Squadron of Baltimores did not like the idea of having an extra member joining their crews, however much he prided himself as an air-gunner. This was because the Baltimore was a small aircraft with very little room in which to move about'.

However, Jimmy remained with the squadron, operating also with the Americans in Bostons and Mitchells during the Sicilian campaign and the invasion of Italy. He experienced two lucky escapes before the crash on take-off from Taranto in which he was left for dead – until somebody turned over his blackened body and said, 'I think this one's still alive, but he can't possibly live long'.

In his first escape, he baled out of a bomber shot down by anti-aircraft fire among the mountains of central Italy. He very nearly went into the mountains with the aircraft because, not wearing his parachute, he had very little time to look round for a harness. He found it as the plane began to fall out of control, and landed just inside the allied lines. He had been lucky. In his haste he had put the harness on the wrong way round, but had found the ripcord on the opposite side in time. His second escape took place when the American ship in which he was returning to his new base headquarters at Naples was hit by an aerial torpedo attack and he was rescued from the sea.

When Jimmy Wright came to East Grinstead, he recognised the soft, confidence-giving voice of the man helping to send him to sleep in the operating theatre.

Many months earlier, as a young assistant with Technicolor, Jimmy had filmed the wounds of a party of six Guinea Pigs conducted by a Dr Russell Davies to the late Sir Harold Gillies' hospital at Basingstoke, for instructional purposes.

Now Jimmy himself was a Guinea Pig and it was the beginning of a long association with Russell Davies who, as medical liaison officer of the Guinea Pig Club and consultant anaesthetist to the Queen Victoria Hospital, is one of the best friends every Guinea Pig has.

# CHAPTER THREE

'Allied to Blackie's monumental labours . . . has been the work of Dr Russell Davies who has developed the uncanny capacity for handling pension cases.'

On a wartime night when overhead the searchlight batteries between London and the coast were handing German raiders on from Sussex-by-the-sea to the Serpentine, Dr Russell Davies could not get off to sleep at East Grinstead. Patients tend to presume a monopoly of insomnia but doctors can worry themselves into sleeplessness too. Even anaesthetists.

The worry which was keeping Russell Davies awake was one which derived not from his professional responsibilities for the Guinea Pigs as one of their anaesthetists but from his humanitarian concern for their future welfare. He was puzzled by the perplexing vagaries of the disability pensions which were beginning to be awarded. How, for example, had the official mind arrived at an award of 92 per cent for Henry Standen, grossly mutilated and with only the sight of half an eye remaining to him in a fearfully disfigured face? Why 92 per cent? Why the 2 per cent? Why not 88 per cent or 96 per cent? Why had a Pig who had lost *one* eye been awarded 40 per cent while Jimmy Wright, sightless in both eyes, rated 100 per cent? The questions kept Russell awake. He got out of bed, drew the blackout curtains and began to write down his first thoughts on Guinea Pigs and pensions. He has not stopped and today, the correspondence in his Guinea Pig Club filing cabinet contains a formidable collection of pension histories and bears witness to this persistent, methodical man's dogged spare-time pension advocacy on behalf of the Guinea Pigs – a labour which, without fracturing his supremely conscientious professionalism, he could have permitted himself to forego.

Disturbed that sleepless night by the illogical, patternless nature of the government's first pension awards to Ward III's patients, Russell Davies devoted the remaining hours to outlining a schedule designed to guide the award of disability pensions to

34

burned people and other recipients of plastic surgery.

As he worked the doctor visualised many of the disabilities he had encountered at the hospital and assessed them as he believed they should be assessed. It was a long night's work, perhaps the best night's work that any man concerned with the welfare of wounded service people has ever done. By morning Russell Davies had arrived at what he believed to be a fair and reasonable guide to the assessment of pension awards for some of the many permutations of disablement. Fairer, certainly, than the schedule of which a pensions official had told him conversationally, 'Roughly speaking, we say fifty per cent for half an injured face and one hundred per cent for a whole injured face and start from there!'

The pensions people had no scale for Guinea Pigs and Russell Davies deduced, therefore, that the Pigs were encountering a rough-and-ready assessment.

Having seen men on the operating table who were having new eyelids fashioned from the soft skin under their arms and at the the same time losing a leg – to give but one example of the many permutations of disablement in the club – Russell Davies was determined to 'sell' his belief that some of the airmen were so badly injured that a maximum rating of 100 per cent was not sufficient.

That night, Russell Davies rated the worst cases at 170 per cent and worked from that basis, with the result that over the years the Guinea Pig Club has managed to obtain the maximum of 100 per cent for men who previously might have rated less than 100 per cent, say, 92 per cent like Henry Standen.

In consequence of Russell's work the club was able to begin its battle, 'to end', as Blackie characteristically insists, 'any such nonsense as any one-eyed member receiving less than 100 per cent disability pension.'

No punches were pulled in this pensions battle. 'To settle matters', Blackie remembers, 'Archie took a top official to the Savage Club. "Agree to our ratings," he said, "or I'll send them back and back again to you and kick up hell in the House".' On another occasion, McIndoe wrote to Blackie, 'I have written to the Ministry re the pensions and am arranging an interview so that we can stop this fantastic nonsense of giving Jock Morris 50 per cent pension and cutting Ross Stewart's pension down to 70 per cent. . . . If they remain bloodyminded, you and Sir Ian

35

Fraser can scare the political daylights out of the . . .'.

The club's success in the pensions' battle has not meant, however, that men as mutilated as Jimmy Wright have received a 170 per cent disability pension. Authority always withstood McIndoe's pressure for the *official* acceptance of Russell Davies's scale, which included what the Guinea Pig Club terms, 'social disability'. But, the club is comforted that the pensions people were quietly relieved to resort to the guidance of Russell's ratings, supported as they were in the beginning by a verbal bombardment, in which the Boss assailed Whitehall with salvoes of New Zealand invective and the despatch from East Grinstead of six 'guinea pig' Guinea Pigs – McIndoe's idea – to test authority's professed intention to improve the early pension awards.

Thenceforth the disability pensions of members of the club were awarded with a more progressive attitude and since that first wartime offensive, Russell's patient reasoning, in case after case, has created a pensions patent for Guinea Pigs. It has also, by its example, assisted the less fortunate, but as badly wounded, men from the Navy and the Army, who are not represented by such a strong 'union' as the Guinea Pig Club.

The Boss missed no opportunity of reminding Pigs of this 'trade union' function of their club. As the years passed, he increased the emphasis which annually, he placed upon his speeches at the Dinner and in 1956, he told the club, 'Most of the Guinea Pigs are doing nicely, apart from such things as the credit squeeze and overdrafts – although we do occasionally get the odd panic telephone call to say that the bums are in, please do something.

'The whole point is that you should stick together and no power on earth can hurt you. *Drift apart – and you've had it!*'

Appealing to the Pigs to help him maintain the active membership of their union, he had said earlier, 'You will probably know the men I mean and I ask you to reach out a hand and drag them back to the fold so that we may try to help them.'

McIndoe was a master at keeping contact without necessarily seeing people. He toiled at the correspondence with which he kept in touch with his Pigs. Sometimes it took not a hand but a very long arm indeed to reach out to a Pig as removed from his 'sty' as René Marchecourt on Rangiroa Island, Tahiti, in the French Society Islands. But the Boss corresponded with René, who remained remembered, 'fifty miles', as he wrote, 'from Tahiti. Quite a lonely place. Just an atoll with a big lagoon in the middle where I am looking after my family coco-nuts'.

* * *

The full measure of Russell's devotion to the Guinea Pigs is known only to the committee of the club and to those Guinea Pigs who have been helped by him. It is very possible that of the approaching 450 thought-to-be surviving members of Pigs who passed through East Grinstead, there are some who are *not* 'doing nicely': who need assistance but are unaware of the help or advice the club can give them, especially of the effect of a letter from Russell Davies or Edward Blacksell.

Sadly, neither the name on the letterhead nor the implied wrath of Sir Archibald McIndoe can be employed any longer but when Prince Phillip willingly accepted Presidency of the Guinea Pig Club, the Pigs were delighted. While, obviously, no attempt would be made to associate the new President with any problem of negotiation, the Guinea Pigs are comforted by the knowledge that neither the Prince nor authority takes lightly any good cause with which he is associated.

Russell's continuing pressure to improve the disability pensions of certain Pigs who will need more help as they grow older, is coupled with his efforts to save others from the cuts which the nation, defaulting on its wartime debt to these airmen, attempts to impose from time to time.

Over the years since their pensions were so terrifyingly earned, the pensions ministry has sought periodically to reduce some Guinea Pig disability pensions. Russell will receive a call, 'I've been told to report for a pension board. What shall I say?' Russell invites the Pig to meet him and they go through all the relevant papers. There are occasions where a cut seems fair and Russell will advise the Pig to accept it. But if in his long experience Russell feels that the club should not countenance the cut, then the old fight is on again.

One of the more callous pieces of official inhumanity the club has had to combat began with a few words on an R.A.F. noticeboard. Without being vouchsafed so much as the privacy of a little buff envelope, Pilot Michael E. Forster, who had flown Lancasters during the war, re-enlisted in the R.A.F.V.R. in 1949 and crashed three months later, read, '2606095 P.II Pilot Forster, M. E. Discharged from the R.A.F.V.R. on 1.3.50. Below the standard required for Air Force Service as a pilot'.

Those last words bit into this badly burned man who had returned to the Air Force from civilian life. 'I might have been discharged because I couldn't make the grade as a pilot and not for medical reasons due to the crash', he told the club. 'I am now in a bit of a state as I am trying to live on 26 shillings a week from National Health. What shall I do?'

In the accident Forster had sustained a compound fracture of the left ankle, a fractured left cheekbone, injury to the spine and multiple burns on face, neck, left arm, both hands, left leg, right knee and both feet. The club fought and obtained Pig Forster's 100 per cent disability pension, with the relevant backdating.

Guinea Pig Peter Brooke had been extensively burned, lost a hand and suffered multiple fractures, including a fracture of the spine. Few men could have been more distressingly injured and disfigured in the defence of his country than this airman. He was awarded a 100 per cent disability pension. One would have supposed that the authorities would have been pleased to leave Peter's award at 100 per cent for the remainder of his life but not long after the award, they began to harry him with nasty little buff envelopes, in which he was informed curtly that his disability pension was being reduced by 10 per cent. The club, the 'trade union', went into action. Russell Davies prepared a pensions brief and the Boss wrote to the Pensions Ministry, 'This very gallant ex-member of aircrew received the most devastating injuries on May 8th, 1942, in action against Germany'. Four months later, the battle won, the surgeon was enabled to write to his Pig, 'My dear Peter, I am delighted to hear that the Ministry have repented and that all is well. If you have any further trouble with these gents, let me know'.

Despite the 'uncanny capacity' Russell Davies has developed for dealing with 'these gents', it is understandable that there are many Pigs who may be in need of his advice and are unaware of his continuing concern for their welfare – particularly the far flung Pigs in Canada, Australia, and New Zealand.

People tend to remember old, but geographically distant friends as they knew them at their height of their association and fail to envisage them as they have become. Thus many Pigs will remember Russell Davies as they found him, a young doctor who had specialised in anaesthetics and who was not much older than most of his patients. They will remember him as a Celtically good looking, young Welsh doctor, rather self-conscious in their company when they were wearing uniform because of his civilian

38

tweed coat and grey flannel trousers. A young doctor who was already a craftsman in what his patients termed the 'knock-out trade', but who was overshadowed by the bulky eminence of their great favourite, Dr John Hunter, the 'Pass Out King' – to whom, as they saw it, Russell compared as an able 'Pass Out apprentice'. This is an appraisal which physical comparison between John Hunter and Russell Davies accentuated. The two anaesthetists were men of contrast. John was 'The Giant Killer' – he was a man of nicknames – with a rollicking joviality and a gargantuan public-house thirst. Russell was slight, diffident and deep.

John died before the Boss. He had needed money to satisfy the demands of his expansive and generous personality and he made it in private practice as McIndoe's anaesthetist. He spent it as quickly as it came, much of it on parties for recuperating Pigs, vast rounds of drinks in the Pig locals and ceaseless hospitality in support of a flow of well told funny stories.

Often his drinking companions would be Pigs due for the 'slab' and John Hunter's 'official' anaesthetic the following day. For these Pigs, the anaesthetist would frown upon spirits. Whisky, gin and rum as it was explained to the patients in lay terms, would send the blood through their veins faster than beer. So John tried to keep them on beer the night before a 'slabbing'. The jester to the Guinea Pig Club, John Hunter, remained alive until the phase of drink and parties and the drowning of inhibitions had passed into the phase of job-finding, educational assistance, loans and grants and hard bargaining for pensions, for which Russell Davies was the more suitable advocate and mediator. When he died, a spray of cream carnations from the Guinea Pig Club lay on his coffin and the card which accompanied the flowers bade farewell to John Hunter and carried a message which will perpetuate the true perspective of the relationship between the Guinea Pigs and their beloved 'Pass Out King':

'In loving memory of and with great regret of Our John of the enormous heart from Guinea Pigs all over the world.'

After John Hunter's death, Russell Davies refused McIndoe's invitation to join him as his anaesthetist in private practice. He gave as his reason his principle that a doctor should work either privately or for the health service but not for both.

Modestly, Russell will not endorse this opinion but undoubtedly there was another reason which partly influenced his decision to remain whole-time at East Grinstead. While he was at the Queen Victoria Hospital, all the Guinea Pigs would know that, despite the passing of time, there would be somebody always there, always at 'the Sty', who knew them, understood their eccentricities and their problems. Russell Davies does accept, however, that had it not been for the Guinea Pigs, he would not have remained at the hospital but would have sought to return to a teaching hospital in London. Therefore, in a manner which would never have occurred to those early Maxillonians, their 'grogging club' was to assist the little cottage hospital of East Grinstead to grow up into the teaching hospital it is becoming.

There are so many and varied examples of this man's after-care and consideration that one finds it difficult to select from them. There is, however, one example which illustrates the delicacy of touch such advocacy can demand. It concerns Flying-Officer Cyril Harper who crash-landed in the Malayan jungle after the war and subsequently, with the help of the club, qualified as an optician.

The most interesting aspect of Cyril Harper's story is that the main problem was not one which is generally taken into account when welfare and benevolent bodies survey a shattered service-man's case. It was, however, by the very nature of the club's general rule that members should have served as aircrew, a problem which was common in the experience of the Guinea Pig Club. Simply, that Cyril Harper like so many young men who were commissioned as aircrew, had bettered himself through the opportunity which his Service career presented.

Ordinarily, had a whole, unbattered Harper returned to civilian life, it was possible that the initiative he had displayed in the Air Force might have taken him ahead in a peacetime career. But, as a disabled Guinea Pig, he faced more than his fair share of hardship if he was to lift himself out of the railway station booking office, where he had been a junior clerk.

The helping of Harper required a finely balanced juggling of the resources from which the club could draw and here Russell played his part. He knew that, because the R.A.F. Benevolent Fund was constituted to meet distress but never wholly to aid self-betterment, that he could not seek complete assistance there for the financing of Harper while he studied for his British Optical Association Diploma. He knew that Harper had one cherished possession – a car. But he also knew that if Harper could show the sacrifice of parting with his car to help pay his way towards professional acceptance as an optician, such sacrifice would impress the Royal Air Force Benevolent Fund and the committee of the Guinea Pig Club.

Cyril Harper sold his car, although this meant that he could not get about very easily as his injuries prevented him walking very far or very well. This money provided one third of the sum he needed to see him through to his Diploma – if he passed the exams. The Benevolent Fund contributed another third and the Club made up the difference. Cyril Harper, former railway clerk, former Flying-Officer became an optician.

\* \* \*

Mainly through his negotiations on behalf of Ian – 'Jock' – Craig who, true Scotsman, put his burns to work as a successful salesman of fire insurance, Russell Davies has developed, in passing, a sideline reputation among Guinea Pigs for negotiating glass eyes.

Jock Craig will tell the tale of his No. 9 glass eye but in common with all Guinea Pigs he prefers not to dwell on the fire which burned away the right side of his face. 'We do not reminisce', Geoff Page reminds Pigs at the Dinners and Blackie says, 'Reminiscence deeper than the schoolboy humour of the Sty recalls horror to some Pigs and is the negation of the euphoric world of guinea piggery into which Archie delivered them'.

This much, however, Jock Craig will say and if it sounds matter-of-fact, then it is because that is the way he tells the story, 'Our bomber was returning to the station when it caught a wing in a balloon cable and plunged towards a bomb dump. I remember after the impact that I instinctively grabbed for my axe but it wasn't there. I made my way through the flames to the nose. Not a soul was there. No pilot. No front gunner. I worked aft again. The flames parted and I saw the ground. I jumped and then I ran and I ran and I ran, chased by rescuers. They caught me and tore my clothes off. I remember thinking that I had been No. 13 at my initial medical and No. 13 when I flew solo. Then, as my tunic was ripped to pieces, I thought of my Observer's wing on the breast pocket. 'Save that brevet', I shouted. 'It cost me four shillings.'

Jock switches, by-passing the years in hospital, the many operations and talks about that glass eye, 'Very disconcerting to find oneself on the point of selling some fire insurance and then out pops the glass eye, bounces off the client's desk and on to the floor. The trouble was that once having accepted a government glass eye, it was not easy to arrange to try out an alternative'.

After considerable correspondence, seven possible substitute glass eyes were despatched to Jock on approval from the Ministry of Pensions. The canny Craig retained two, one to wear, one as a spare, never thinking that the extra eye would call for the advice and intervention of the Guinea Pig Club through the medium of the medical liaison officer, Russell Davies.

The Ministry, it appeared, could not understand what practical use a one-glass-eyed man could possibly make of two government glass eyes. All Jock sought was the security of knowing that he carried a spare eye in his wallet.

At the conclusion of the correspondence and after more cost in time and postage than the price of the eye, which with his native sense of good husbandry he had retained, Jock Craig was allowed to keep the spare eye. But only after a special authority – one No. 9 eye, Craig for the use of – had been obtained from the Air Ministry.

\* \* \*

The Guinea Pig Club, and in this connection the club means mainly Russell Davies, has been helped substantially when presenting pension claims by the Pigs' personal knowledge of their medical and surgical history. At the risk of creating a host of hospital bores (which up to a point he did!) McIndoe encouraged Pig patients to understand their operations. His patience in explaining each step to each patient proved a morale maker, like good relations between enlightened management and the men and women on the factory floor. And it served practical purposes. One finds former Flight-Lieutenant Laurence Chiswell writing, 'Although I am supposed to be finished, perhaps sometime you could drop my top lip on the left side which, as I pointed out at the last Guinea Pig week-end, has shrunk again somewhat since it was done three years ago.'

During the war Richard Hillary employed the knowledge he had gained so painfully at the Sty to help Britain at the highest diplomatic level in the United States. His problem was that after arriving in America to lecture and broadcast during the summer of 1941, British Embassy officials complained that he was too horrific in appearance. His plastic surgery was incomplete and the diplomatists took the view that Hillary could do more harm than good by appearing like that, in an America which Winston Churchill was hoping to bring into the war.

Chagrined by this attitude, the young fighter pilot cabled McIndoe for permission to be operated upon by Dr Jerome Webster at the New York Medical Center. At the same time, at Hillary's request, Duff Cooper, Britain's Ambassador to Washington, cabled Sir Archibald Sinclair, the Liberal Air Minister in Churchill's wartime government, for his blessing on Hillary's activities.

Hillary was 'slabbed', as Guinea Pigs say, and afterwards he wrote to McIndoe, 'I have to confess that I persuaded Webster considerably against his will, to do a graft over the bridge of my nose between my eyes. I did this partly as a sop to official Washington which, as you may know, had been yammering for me to have my face done and partly because there has been some contraction of my left lower lid. My face is actually improved but as our officials here have such a bee in their bonnet about it, I doubt if they could ever be persuaded to notice the face unless I had some little job done.'

The Pigs visited the operating theatres more frequently as observers than as patients and improved the knowledge gained from discussion of their own operations by watching the plastic surgeons at work on their friends. It is, as every addict of hospital serials on television will appreciate, not the usual practice in hospitals to allow patients to wander in and out of the operating theatres, wearing dressing gowns. There was little that was usual about the Sty. Relatives like Jimmy Wright's father, who watched operations on his son from over McIndoe's shoulder were welcome too.

George Taylor, who built up a successful motor car agency in New South Wales, was one of the most badly injured among the happy fraternity of Australian Pigs. He comments, 'Through watching many different types of plastic surgery operations some of the Pigs learned to be very selective when discussing with their surgeons the types of grafts they wanted. In the latter stages the Boss used to allow me to write down the various jobs I wanted performed, so that we could talk over the list, discussing such things as whether I should have the Thiersch, Dermatome or Epidermoplasty between the fingers: or the merits or demerits of Wolfe, Full Thickness, Partial Thickness, or Dermatome on the palms of the hands. He would sometimes indicate why a flap graft in a particular position would do the best job but why

43

another type as compromise would be better because of the time factor.

'There was no such thing as saying, "Who's doing this job? You leave it to me!" On the contrary, he would treat those Air Force patients who chose to be interested, as though they were a paying clientele with a competitive choice and seek their opinions as plainly as a shoe shop salesman.'

After such consultations, George Taylor and his friends made out what they called their 'shopping list' and pinned it to the fronts of their operation smocks before being wheeled into the theatre. George's list always started with which hand he wished to be done. This was because he had had it agreed with the Boss that once the hands were healed and beginning to be useful, it would be a calamity if, following an operation on both hands at once for the purpose of gaining extra movement, he contracted an infection in both hands simultaneously. Like men who have wobbled on the tightrope of financial disaster, the mutilated learn that it is wise to keep a reserve. A Guinea Pig rediscovering the use of one hand after weeks of dependence, counted himself a veritable Lord of the Sty. One needed a free hand, in any event, to grope for the shopping list upon surfacing from the anaesthetic. Each completed item would be neatly ticked and against the unfinished jobs, the surgeon had noted appropriate comments and explanations.

Familiarity invariably produces awkward situations. This intimate relationship between surgeons and patients proved a magnificent morale builder but it led to one especially delicate problem. Individual Pigs grew rather choosy about their surgeons. They recognised certain surgeons as being more skilled, say, at hands than noses, at eyelids than legs and they put themselves down for operations by specified surgeons, in accordance with a personal assessment of their abilities.

Much discussion of the surgeons and of their talents took place in the wards and in the public houses of East Grinstead and generally, the surgeons accepted it in good spirit. From time to time, however, visiting surgeons encountered an openly hostile distrust among their patients – and the perplexing phenomenon of a surgically astute pilot, navigator or air-gunner presenting his shopping list!

There was, however, sufficient psychological and practical benefit to neutralise the occasional awkward situation and in time, the medical profession was to benefit from this unusual practice. A number of Pigs subsequently engaged themselves in medicine, including Tommy Brandon, who became the senior medical photographer at St Thomas' Hospital, and Bertram Owen-Smith who, helped by the club and personal encouragement from Russell Davies and the Boss, became a plastic surgeon.

Moreover, as has been indicated the Pig's unorthodox relationship with the Sty's medical staff, was to prove helpful in the pensions' war.

Appearing before a tribunal, John Taylor, suspecting that the club's case that his stomach ulcer was attributable to his R.A.F. service, was not going too well, fumbled in his pocket. With that touch of theatre, which guinea piggery seems to bestow upon most of those associated with it, he produced and explained the relevant and pickled portion of his inside.

# CHAPTER FOUR

'As we worked a persistent question nagged at my mind: when their bodies are whole again can we also rebuild something of their lives?'

Bertram Owen-Smith left school at seventeen and a half and worked in an estate agent's office for six months until he was old enough to begin his training as a pilot. He did not possess the school certificate when the Air Force accepted him but he worked hard and was an operational pilot when the accident happened in which he lost a great deal of his face. His hands were burned too, but not beyond repair, and the surgical skill of McIndoe and his team enabled him to return to operational flying between surgical operations. A number of the Pigs indulged in this somewhat aggressive form of occupational therapy and at those stages in the war when operationally trained aircrew were in small supply, the country was grateful for the resumed services of a half-repaired, semi-fried Guinea Pig. Some of the Pigs, like Geoff Page and the Czech fighter pilot, Frankie Truhlar, their first repairs incomplete, returned to the Sty with new wounds.

Nevertheless, there were many long weeks when a Pig had to lie in a ward and wait and it was during these weeks that Bertram Owen-Smith, the young estate agent's clerk from Swansea, nourished an ambition – to become a plastic surgeon. He educated himself in bed and matriculated at the Sty. Nobody in the club thought he would ever qualify as a doctor and then as a surgeon. But the club stuck to its great principle that a Pig with an ambition should be given every opportunity to prove to himself that he could not fulfil it. Financial help was provided. Owen-Smith became a doctor and a surgeon, worked under McIndoe at East Grinstead and eventually a leading consultant in plastic surgery in southern Africa.

Those early Maxillonians in Ward III would have raised an unbelieving roar, had anybody suggested that their 'grogging club' would help to find the means for paying the way for a future plastic surgeon from among the Guinea Pigs or that they would provide from among their number, doctors, opticians, sanitary inspectors, accountants and trained men in many professions. Had there not been, as will be recalled, some difficulty in finding a pair of hands to uncork and pour the sherry on that sunny Sunday morning in 1941?

It is certain, therefore, that the roar of disbelief would have been heightened had anybody added *forestry* to the list of future Guinea Pig occupations.

Nobody at the Queen Victoria Hospital really believed that J.D. would one day stand before a tree with an axe in his hands. He had no fingers with which to grip the handle of an axe. If you clench your fists and look down at your knuckles, you will gain some understanding of what remained to J.D. of his hands. You may also agree with what even the Maestro accepted at the time – that in applying to J.D. the guiding principle of allowing a Pig to discover for himself that he could not fulfil his ambition, the Guinea Pig Club would be encouraging the impossible.

From his bed, J.D. told the surgeon, 'I would like to become a forester'. McIndoe replied, 'I will do my best but it will necessitate additional operations on your hands and even then I cannot promise you that you will be able to hold an axe'.

The great principle was to be put to the test, irrespective of the cost in time and money. Nevertheless, if it comforted the young Scot, who had come from his 15s. 0d. a week job as a village draper's assistant, to fly with the Air Force, to face a long series of surgical operations with a dream of great trees falling to his axe, then it was desirable that this flicker of hope be allowed him.

If you look at your fist again and feel down the top of your hands from the knuckle of each finger, you will discover something of which hitherto you may not have been conscious. Your fingers begin near the wrist. When McIndoe told J.D. he would have to undergo additional operations, he had conceived the idea of contriving artificial clefts in the palms of the patient's hands. The operations took place. At intervals between them, McIndoe arranged for Jock to visit a forestry estate in Gloucestershire and to begin to get the feel of an axe, starting with a light five pounder.

The result was a successful and jubilant J.D. He married his nurse who was a South African girl and soon Russell Davies was writing to the Burns Committee of the R.A.F. Benevolent Fund, 'It was the opinion of everybody who met him that physically J.D. would be unable to do manual labour in the open

47

air by virtue of his extremely serious burns with residual scarring of both face and hands. However, it was felt that he should be allowed to follow his inclination in order that he could prove to himself that he was unable to fulfil his wishes'.

In 1950, J.D. and his wife, with the help of the club, sailed for South Africa. The rest of their story is not so happy, partly one suspects because once in South Africa, J.D. was beyond the reach of the regular assurance and encouragement of Blackie and Russell.

At first, however, they seemed to be happy. J.D. wrote to the club, 'I am very keen to settle here. The climate seems ideal for Guinea Pigs.' But it did not take long for another aspect of South Africa to dispirit him. Wielding an axe was a coloured man's job. Employers did not put it to Jock exactly in this way and like so many manual workers who labour alongside coloured men in Britain, it would not have concerned him. But whenever he applied for a manual job in forestry his 'mitts', as he reported to the club, were viewed without sympathy.

When, eventually, he found work with a wool firm, it was not in the open air as he had hoped. He was, as a white man must be in the Union of South Africa, an overseer of coloured labour. A wool slump put him out of work and the ensuing uncertainty which would have been distressing enough to an uninjured man disturbed J.D.'s peace of mind. The Guinea Pig Club, watching with concern from a distance, was relieved when news arrived that he had found a new job in an oxygen plant. Unfortunately, he could not hold it down and when he left he deteriorated mentally.

J.D.'s parents made the long voyage from Scotland to the Cape to see their son and expressed their opinion to the club that if he returned home he would be restored to normal mental health. Local medical opinion disagreed. J.D. was schizophrenic and dangerous, it was reported.

This medical report confronted the club with a distressing dilemma and one of the last of McIndoe's actions on behalf of any of his Pigs was to examine J.D.'s case with Russell Davies.

The facts were that if the club decided to find the money to bring J.D. home – and this would have been very expensive because air travel and two male attendants were being insisted upon by the South African authorities – then he would be separated from his wife and two children, perhaps forever. She was willing to let J.D. go if it was considered by McIndoe to be in his best interest but she felt that she should stay in South Africa bring up the children. Her family and roots were there.

J.D. never returned to Scotland. He was beyond decision on his own behalf and the club decided that it would be better for him to be near his wife and family. He remained, withdrawn and solitary, in a South African mental hospital. Possibly the courage of the young Scottish shop assistant who went to war and accepted those additional operations in order to equip himself to earn a living as a forester, expended its final reserve when he was sacked by the wool firm just before his fortieth birthday. Possibly, there was – as Russell Davies believes – an underlying tendency towards schizophrenia. Certainly, there is no question but that J.D.'s sad history upholds the wisdom of those British-born Pigs who fear to venture too far from Barnstaple or East Grinstead.

The Guinea Pig Club kept in touch with his wife and helped her to educate her Piglet children. She worked in Pretoria, a nurse again, as she was when she tended the Pigs at the Sty and met J.D.

* * *

Bill Foxley's body will never be whole again. He can see, but with less than Nelson at Trafalgar. He carries one glinting, well polished, meticulously matched glass eye in the right socket and sight only remains in one half of his left eye. He has a new, expressionless face, in which the most animate feature is the glass eye when the light catches it. His face is emotionless because fire destroyed skin, muscle, everything facial up to the eyebrows with which Bill Foxley arrived in this world.

Surgeons can graft skin to cover the blackened, contracted mess of a man's face but they cannot simulate so much as a puppet's smile. They leave, as with some of the Guinea Pigs, a static clown-like grin.

Bill Foxley's emotions, then, cannot be observed in the eyes or in the face. Nor can they be detected in the hands. Bill has no hands. But they are expressed, none the less, by the agitation of the scarred stumps which end where whole men's hands begin and by an increased rate of blink of his reconstructed eyelids.

When Bill Foxley dies he will not look his age. The youthful high spirits with which he sallied into aircrew have not left him and surgery has rendered him facially ageless. Only his greying hair betray the advancing years. When one considers this man's injuries, one immediately understands why even Blackie, the great optimist, feared that the club would have to face the prospect that Bill Foxley would be unemployable.

Bill Foxley became the house manager for a large Central Electricity Generating Board building.

McIndoe was to say, 'As we worked, a persistent question nagged at my mind: when their bodies are whole again can we also rebuild something of their shattered lives? *Something* of Bill Foxley's shattered life *has been* rebuilt – but only after years of endeavour on his own behalf and on that of the Guinea Pig Club.

Reconstruction of his face nearing completion, Bill's high spirits persuaded him and those responsible for his welfare that, in common with many Pigs, while he may have been maimed and disfigured, he remained a fit man.

Bill Foxley's body was as whole again as McIndoe and his surgeons could make it and he set out to show how fit a Guinea Pig could become. He went into athletic training, creating a fair reputation for himself as a runner before the years, which are not apparent, began to slow him down. He also married Cath, a very attractive East Grinstead girl who had worked in the Hospital Treasurer's office.

In passing, Bill was not alone among Guinea Pigs who subsequently excelled in sport. The club's membership included former Flight-Lieutenant 'Kim' Hall, a golf professional and another Flight-Lieutenant, Bob Graham, who having lost his eye and his right arm in a 1941 night flying accident, won the one-armed golf championship ten years later. Bertram Owen-Smith played rugger for Westminster Hospital.

Athletic though he was, Bill Foxley's physical fitness was of little avail to him when he returned to his work in an ironmonger's shop. Fumbling for the nails and other sharp articles which are inevitable to that trade, the stumpy remains of his hands began to bleed.

Here Blackie came into the picture and because sweets and tobacco are easier to handle than nails and nuts and bolts, Bill was helped to establish himself in Boutport Street, not many minutes from Blackie's home at Barnstaple.

Bill and Cath worked hard at shopkeeping but even Bill will admit that he was not nature's shopkeeper and in time the club decided to help Bill out of his shop and into a new occupation. Before the final decision to make a change a small incident happened which, because of its smallness, reveals and records the debt the Guinea Pig Club owes to Air Vice-Marshal Sir John Cordingley, late Controller of the Royal Air Force Benevolent Fund, for his affection and unflagging personal interest in its members' individual affairs. Sir John called on Bill's shop in Barnstaple and sensed that, with increased competition, all was not as well as it had been when controls were still in force and Bill was receiving good supplies. For in the early days of peace, one of the club's most useful services for its shopkeeping members was to alleviate the problems of shortage. Thus, for instance, Blackie was to write to a toffee manufacturer on behalf of Bill, 'I wonder if you can help this man by increasing his allocation of toffees. I can assure you that if you can manage this you will be assisting a most deserving man to take his place in the community again and in spite of his gross injuries to be an economic asset to the town in which he lives'.

When Bill left the shop even Blackie worried privately that, with only half an eye, Bill might have to be accepted as unemployable, apart possibly from mouldering in one of the financially and mentally unrewarding jobs usually available to disabled men.

But, such is the spirit of guinea-piggery, that former Warrant Officer Bill Foxley has commuted daily between Crawley and London for his work with the Central Electricity Generating Board. Nearby, a retired and whole Air Commodore held a similar position.

It was another Pig, Sam Gallop, an editor of the Guinea Pig magazine and a Deputy Secretary of the Central Electricity Generating Board, who helped Bill into the career for which he has proved himself as suited, if not more suited, than many whole men.

Sam first encountered Bill in 1943 when they occupied adjacent beds at East Grinstead. Bill was enveloped in white bandages. 'The invisible man himself,' Sam thought, 'and then a voice emerged and revealed to me the important fact, "you can get eggs here." '

While Sam Gallop was at the hospital he never saw Bill. Only 'the invisible man'. In 1945 they were introduced at a party as strangers, and then they discovered that they knew each other. Later Sam heard about Bill's difficulties and visited him in Barnstaple. Sam provided him with the opportunity of an interview. 'Since that time he has been doing a magnificent job', Sam says, 'and has been promoted on merit'.

Several Guinea Pigs became doctors, but there is only one doctor who became a Guinea Pig. Owen-Smith's hands were repaired so that he could operate as a plastic surgeon when he had qualified. Noel Newman, an R.A.F. doctor, looked at his hands after the flames had roasted them in a desert air crash, and knew that the fire had robbed him of all opportunity to become an orthopaedic surgeon as he had wished.

That he was a doctor did not spare 'Doc' Newman from experiencing many of the same fears and misgivings of his fellow Pigs. But he *was* a Pig with a difference. He found himself urged by his professional training to seek to investigate his recovery rather than to drown it. He said, 'When you are first injured, and if in pain, you hope to die. As soon as the drugs become effective or the pain eases, you hope to live. The smallest things begin to become something to live for. Even if it's only the Irish stew for lunch. Then you begin to take the small things for granted and the process continues.'

At this point, Newman discovered, many pigs – including himself – approached their greatest crisis. 'After weeks, perhaps months, of pampering somebody says, "Do it yourself". The spoiling is over. You are reckoned well enough to begin to do little chores for yourself. And then you find you cannot do them, or they take patience and cause pain. Very ordinary functions which men take for granted. Shoe laces. Fly buttons. Tooth brushing. Even sipping a glass of beer in bed. The distress at this point is savage, and few are the Pigs whose pillows were not stained by tears of bitterness.'

'Doc' Newman believes that there are Pigs who never overcame the crisis point and that they are to be found amongst those who remain most in need of the club, though some of them may not have remained closely in touch with it.

\* \* \*

Few members of the club rebuilt their lives in the air but among their very small number is a survivor from a blazing Spitfire, Jackie Mann. He later captained airliners. 'I feel that I am, perhaps, unique among Guinea Pigs', he said, and this was not because he was an airline captain. Jackie Mann photographed his fighter plane immediately after it had hit the ground – or as he says, 'I photographed my own birth as a Pig'.

Jack Mann was shot down five times before he received the burns which qualified him for membership of the club. On the fourth occasion – it was late in the afternoon of September 14th, 1940 (and thus on the eve of the great day of battles fought between London and the south coast) – his parents were told he was dead and arrived at the hospital with a coffin to receive his remains.

The mortuary keeper told Sergeant Mann's father, 'We have several pilots here and we don't know which of them is your son. Nobody would be able to tell. Frankly we don't mind which one you take.'

Mr Mann felt that perhaps the police sergeant who had accompanied the body to the hospital could assure identification and called on him. From the sergeant he learned there had been a mistake. His son was alive and in the hospital.

On not one of his six crashes did Jack Mann bale out. In each case he crash-landed his fighter and, although he regrets missing the experience of a parachute descent, he observed one descent which he will never forget. He had circled protectingly round a pilot who had baled out and whose body was on fire. At 1,000 feet the pilot suddenly dropped clear of his parachute harness. Whether he released himself or whether the fire had burned him out of the harness, Jack never discovered. But at the moment the airman's body fell away to the ground one thousand feet below, black smoke was curling up from his seat, up his back and round his neck. One of many airmen who did not live to become a Guinea Pig.

Twenty-one years afterwards, Jack Mann, a Comet Captain with Middle East Airlines wrote to Tom Gleave, 'That I have reason to be grateful, oh inadequate word, to Archie McIndoe, is readily evident from the following quotation from "Tally Ho!" (Yankee in a Spitfire) by Arthur Gerald Donahue; the Macmillan Company, New York, 1941:

'Two of the boys had been badly wounded and at least one of them, Sergeant Mann, is not expected to fly again. He was awarded the Distinguished Flying Medal while in the hospital. This boy had been shot down for the sixth time. His machine was badly shot up and his engine wrecked over the Channel but he managed to glide back over land. Then, when he was only two hundred feet up, too low to bale out, his machine caught fire and he had to force land it in a farmer's field. He crawled out of the cockpit then and in spite of the fact that he was terribly burned, he took his camera out of his pocket, carefully adjusted it for light and distance and snapped the pictures of the blazing wreck, after which he staggered across two fields to the farm house."'

Captain Jack Mann continued his letter to the Chief Guinea Pig.

'Art Donahue, unfortunately, did not live to see the day the Boss would prove the pundits wrong; at the time of writing, some fifteen thousand flying hours wrong. So much wrong that during this month I expect to start flight conversion on to Comet 4.c.s.'

Recalling his sixth escape, Jack Mann writes, 'On April 4th, 1941, I began the day as a Sergeant Pilot of 91 Squadron, operating from Hawkinge and ended it by being reborn a Guinea Pig in a field at Paddlesworth, Kent, within sight of Hawkinge.

'After some time – days being sightless and timeless – in the Royal Victoria Hospital, Folkstone (I have an idea it was 10–14), I was told I was being removed to East Grinstead.

'In my abysmal ignorance I rebelled at being moved so abruptly from the vicinity of my birthplace but I went – and arrived and into a saline bath. And more saline baths until such time as, fragment by fragment, the suppurating leather skin formed by copious applications of tannic acid, could be cut by scalpel from my legs. And until such time as the scar tissue around my eyes had reached a stage where the Maestro could say, "You are for the slab this morning Jackie". Then my protest, "But my people are coming to see me this morning" and his inimitable response, "Oh, we'll have you back by then" and his instructions to John Hunter, his highly regarded aide and anaesthetist, "Just keep him under, he has visitors coming".'

There are more details of Jack Mann's sixth 'life' and his 're-birth as a Guinea Pig' than appear in the airline Captain's letter to Tom Gleave. Guinea Pigs are reticent about recounting their experiences, particularly to one another, and few Pigs are aware of their fellow Pigs' experiences. If there is one strong inhibition remaining among the majority of members of the Guinea Pig Club, it is an unreadiness to talk about themselves, which derives from fear of appearing to shoot a line. They know of course, of Richard Hillary, Bill Simpson and Richard Pape because they have written their personal stories. And of Paul Hart, the bulb-growing Guinea Pig whom Wilfred Pickles 'advertised' somewhat controversially on the B.B.C. and who has worked well to prosper the opportunity thus presented to him. But of the remainder, they know little excepting such hospital hilarities as the ducking, or attempted ducking, of Sister Meally, of Ward III; or the wheelchair 'chariot' races down the steep hill which leads from East Grinstead towards the foot of the hospital.

Thus, for example, one finds that asked to send the Chief Guinea Pig details of his experiences in and out of hospital, former Flight-Lieutenant Brian Birks, D.F.C. – he was station aircraft safety officer when he walked into a turning propeller – wrote:

'Most memorable experience: Admission to Ward III to the accompaniment of female shrieks and the sight of a battered pyjama-clad patient carrying the immaculately uniformed ward sister towards a bath of cold water.'

Or Jack Toper, subsequently a Marks and Spencer manager, '29th August, 1943. Crash landed Clacton-on-sea (bombs gone of course). D. Day, 1944, saw yours truly sharing a room at Marchwood Park with twenty other types. This was the beginning of doodlebugs. One of the room mates was more than concerned with his second degree burns on his mitts. Came the night. Doodles falling around. Bedroom door closed. A hand handle to turn. We were watching the fireworks. Suddenly a doodlebug cut out above us. There was a mad rush to the door to belt down to the basement. We found (at least two of us did) the door was too difficult to open. We had visions of unpleasant happenings. Lo and behold, the chap with the poor mitts opened the door and we all made our escape. Thereafter, he didn't have a leg to stand on'. The last sentence being underlined by Jack Toper, who continued, 'Following a visit to the slab in conjunction with my rhino pedicle (for the ignoramus, a new nose) was residing in the Canadian wing. The day after I was jissing around the ward with a charming French Canadian Sister, feeling pleased with life at the prospect of a new trunk. That night it was action stations. I had a haemorrhage. The Guinea Pig dinner (1944) was two days away. Yes, I missed it. Blackie commiserated and supplied me with a whole chicken as compensation. When the chicken arrived, to my astonishment, I was the most popular man in the wing. That's right. The types helped me to eat it. They left me the Parson's Nose.'

Francis 'Dixie' Dean, asked for his best rehabilitation story,

wrote 'There were so many! One I recall was while at Marchwood Park. A crowd of us were invited to the local A.T.S. mess for a Do. Lashings of grog and girls. However, towards the end, namely, midnight, "Dixie" was missing. The guards were called out to search all the girls' billets and beds – they knew where to look as they thought. Alas, they could not find me. They did in the end, in an A.T.S. sergeant's bed *ALONE* with a black eye, and to this day, I do not know how I got it – except I've got a photo of an A.T.S. sergeant and written on the back is the following,
"Here's to the aircrew boy with the auburn hair,
Who got a black eye,
Through taking a dare!" '

\*　　\*　　\*

It was late afternoon on the day early in April, 1941, when Jack Mann – who by now, one trusts, stands absolved of any accusation of shooting a line! – crash-landed his Spitfire in flames. Following a report of two enemy aircraft approaching Ramsgate, he had been ordered up from Hawkinge with Sergeant Spears, a nephew of McCudden, fighter ace of the first war. After a while Mann and Spears were told the enemy had gone home. The two pilots relaxed and it was then that the enemy, still very much around, shot Spears down. Jack Mann stopped between ten and fifteen cannon shells. On five previous occasions he had taken his aircraft back, albeit for a crash-landing, and he was determined to return to his airfield again. Just short of Hawkinge his Spitfire started to smoke. He had selected a field for his forced-landing when he noticed that there was a great deal of petrol in the cockpit but by this time his altitude was less than 400 feet. It was too late to bale out. He remembers, 'All I could do was close my eyes and hold the plane as it was going'. The cockpit on fire, Mann made his landing with his eyes tight shut. The starboard wing dropped off on impact – it had been shot up with cannon shell – and killed two sheep.

Then a curious thing happened. Momentarily Jack was convinced that he had landed in occupied country and that he must immediately go through the escape drill. He attributes this to a fear nursed since boyhood of falling prisoner-of-war to the Germans. An uncle had been made prisoner in the first war.

With his clothes on fire and attempting to beat them out, he returned to the cockpit for his parachute and hurled it into a ditch. If the 'enemy' failed to find his parachute, he thought, they would think he had baled out miles away and search elsewhere while he sought friends to help him escape.

Jack started off through two fields and came to a cottage. He was much relieved to find an elderly English woman at the door. She added to his sense of anti-climax. 'I am so sorry you have experienced such a horrid motor cycle accident', she said. Whereupon she fetched her pushbike and rode for a doctor.

A year later Jack Mann was back in the air but in 1943 he received a posting to a ground job in India. He was now married and his wife urgently contacted the Maestro, 'Take him off flying', she said, 'and he'll blow up'. The posting was cancelled and as has been related, Captain Jack Mann of Middle East Airlines carried on flying.

# CHAPTER FIVE

'Social disability is by far the greatest handicap.'

The Guinea Pig Club is registered as an official war charity to obviate taxation. Here, however, in the non-biblical sense of a misused word ends any connection between the club and charity. McIndoe detested the word charity and all the anachronistic nineteenth-century attitudes a conservative-minded British public retains toward it; attitudes which are abetted by the belief, never far below the conscious, that in spite of the welfare state and national insurance, there'll always be an England as long as there are flag days, institutions part-paid by flag days, garden parties, fêtes, and jumble sales.

Charitable organisation in name, then, because an official mentality, awaiting its clockwork M.B.E.s, O.B.E.s, C.B.E.s, and 'K's, would never understand a charitable body which operated a fetish of forbidding charity, the Guinea Pig Club neither canvasses charitable support nor administers a charitable flow in the accepted sense of a word and a process it disdains.

Having, at the Queen Victoria Hospital, as he wrote in the Post-graduate Medical Journal in 1943, 'removed the institutional atmosphere which is the curse of much hospital life', McIndoe called charity his second enemy and worked to save his Pigs from it.

Persistently he sought to divert men from institutions, or from the generally menial and poorly paid jobs allocated to disabled service people, and to launch them into competitive life, knowing that often the physical effort might prove too arduous. Always he insisted, 'Exhaust *all* sources before dealing with the matter as a charity'. Frequently he adjured, 'a Guinea Pig should be a useful member of the community and not playing a cornet in Piccadilly.'

Inevitably, this almost masochistic denial of alms was to compel some of the former airmen into competitive occupations, the stress of which has told, or will tell in time. Rather risk 'charitable' obligations in the future, McIndoe held, than condemn men to unvarying years of enforced helplessness, knitting, rug-making an institutionalised life away, firmly – if kindly – disciplined like the mentally deficient because the burns of war had made them different from those who would keep them in hiding.

McIndoe's creed has endowed the club with a future responsibility which will test it more demandingly than any in the past; responsibility for the Guinea Pigs as they age, or whose disabilities enlarge the usual worries of growing older. Accepting this responsibility, the club is mightily consoled by its favoured relationship with the giant Royal Air Force Benevolent Fund, the fund which Sir Winston Churchill had called, 'part of the conscience of the British nation'. Indeed, Sir Winston, pointedly if unintentionally, forecast the future significance of the fund's intimate accord with the Guinea Pig Club when he broadcast, 'It is our duty now to make sure that the Fund will be able to go on helping, and not fail as the survivors of the war grow old and feeble'.

Growing old and feeble as a Guinea Pig will mean failing sight when you have only half an eye, or if you are more fortunate, one eye; rheumatic 'fingers' on your stumpy hands. Executively such distress is, and will be met, by the decisions of the 'Burns Committee' which connects the 'Ben Fund' and the club and for the work of which the club will ever remain especially indebted to Air Vice-Marshal Sir John Cordingley, a former Controller of the Royal Air Force Benevolent Fund.

One has written that there is no connection between the Guinea Pig Club and charity and then, almost in the same breath that that representations are made to the 'Ben Fund' on behalf of Guinea Pigs. The issue is that there is no connection between the Club and charity as the flag-buying public conceives charity. The 'Ben Fund' is, as Sir Winston said, 'part of the conscience of the British nation'. Whether by loan, or by grant, the cash benefaction is the delayed acknowledgement of former service and sacrifice.

A Guinea Pig fighter pilot, fried in a Spitfire during the Battle of Britain, was privileged to endorse this acknowledgement in the course of an anonymous broadcast Appeal on behalf of the Royal Air Force Benevolent Fund. He said, 'The Battle of Britain meant my facing the fact that I should never use my hands again, and that I was burned and scarred for life. For a time I didn't

59

even want to live. That is what despair does. The R.A.F. Benevolent Fund convinced me that I could start again in a life of my own choosing – and assisted me with means to do it'.

This Guinea Pig who 'didn't want to live' is headmaster of his own private and flourishing preparatory school in Surrey. He is Peter Weeks, the Maxillonian, who as it will be recalled from the beginning of this story, had been elected secretary of the grogging club because, in that moment of hospital hilarity, it seemed appropriate to appoint a secretary who could not write and might never write again.

\* \* \*

There is a distinction between the long-term help the 'Ben' fund can provide from its broad purse and the generally shorter term loans and gifts within the comparatively infinitesimal financial ability of the Guinea Pig Club.

Apart from some larger loans made shortly after the war to propel certain members into commercial or professional life, the club, leaning on the Benevolent Fund for substantial sums, has concentrated upon the provision of first-aid to defeat the depressions of social disability. Here, also, there can be found no definable 'charitable' process through which the Guinea Pig Club holds out a helping hand. Its actions, between the annual 'Lost Weekend' pep mixture of boisterous goodwill, physical, mental and welfare stocktaking and alcoholic bonhomie, are prompted not by any written constitution but by McIndoe's uncompromising dictum, 'Social disability is the greatest handicap'. Twenty-one years after those early Maxillonians met in War III, the club's tiny resources are devoted mainly to reducing that handicap. At times, their employment has been sufficiently exotic to ensure that the spirit of 1940 and 1941 still imbues some of the club's actions and that the club continues to supply a unique service which, with the best will in the world, no rule-ridden 'charitable' organisation could achieve. One wonders, for instance, what 'charity' would accept that a 'course of a week's night-clubbing with plenty of money in his pocket' was the one treatment to return a certain socially disabled man to circulation.

Shocking waste? It worked, and while there can be no proof, it is probable that this enlightened hand-out at the critical moment saved a man from many years in an institution at the expense of the taxpayers for whom he had fought.

Revealing this example of the club's determination to regard every member as a very individual individual, one accepts responsibility for the danger that the telephone operators will be besieged by reversed charge calls from Pigs pleading the headmaster of Barnstaple Secondary Modern for a therapeutic night on the town. But before he reaches for the telephone let any Pig be reminded that over the years such inspired boosts have usually originated from the sixth sense which years of experience of guinea-piggery developed in the brains of the Boss, Russell and Blackie. A fiver here, a case of whisky there. A tenner. A coat for the winter.

'Blackie' to 'Archie' July 25th, 1951: 'You remember the suggestion with regard to X? I am sending form made out for £10 which I should like you to send him with your good wishes to enable him to enjoy a good holiday. I have reason to believe that he would enjoy this more than a case of whisky as I first suggested. Will you write a note that Harvey can send with the cheque?' Today, X flourishes as an executive in an oil company.

'Blackie' to 'Archie' Nov. 27, 1952: 'I have had a long letter from Y explaining the position with regard to his child who, as you may know, was born a Mongol. At the present time he is paying £3.17.6. a week for the child to be boarded out. This is well beyond his income capacity and I think the club will be doing a good job if I send him a cheque for £50.'

Although such acts of *true* charity may seem trivial alongside the club's pension battles, or say, the long-term financing to process an inadequately educated air-gunner into a school-teacher, they have succeeded in renewing confidence when it has reached its lowest mark and have kept men in the competitive world who otherwise might have deteriorated into even more problematical people.

There are, however, more ways of pulling a man up than re-assuring him with kind words and cash handouts and the Guinea Pig Club has never feared to drop the fairy godmother's wand and wield a broad cudgel when ferocity has been considered necessary. But backing the cudgel there has always been kindness.

To a Guinea Pig thrice jailed the Boss would write harshly. To a solicitor about the same man . . . 'I have borne with this young man's troubles for twenty-two years and I do not suppose that we shall ever come to an end of them.'

Then, one finds Blackie blasting another Pig . . . 'we have spent an enormous amount of time and trouble over your re-settlement and it's most depressing to receive an unsatisfactory report of your work with. . . . The impression I gathered was that you are just not putting your back into your work but I am told further that you are hoping to get a grant from the R.A.F. Benevolent Fund to start yourself in a grocery business. Let me say at once that, so bad has been our experience with you in relation to a business of any kind run by yourself, that under no circumstances would I support this application.'

After reminding this Pig of his 'easier opportunity to attain that position of respect in the community which most men who have been through what you have been through do easily command', Blackie wrote a kind letter to the man's firm, hoping that they would bear with him and give him another chance.

One of the legless Pigs was told, 'Pull your socks up, even if they are on tin legs'.

\* \* \*

It is unusual in these times of selfish endeavour, that such a club should have survived the early post-war years. It would not have done so had not those three humanitarians, the Boss, Russell and Blackie remained involved long, long after they could have released themselves from this exacting tie to their duty of the past. Far from making the excuse of new personal and professional responsibilities which would have been understood, the three men deepened the well of their involvement, bringing to Pigs in need that close and personal continuity of assurance and encouragement which is exceptionally fatiguing to the 'giver'.

Bill Foxley's installation on Blackie's doorstep, though it may have been mistaken as his subsequent success with the Central Electricity Generating Board seems to show, demonstrated a measure of the depth of this well.

McIndoe was prepared, without notice, to take a pig into his home. He knew that nearness to the source of confidence could mean the difference between hope and despair to a man not long deprived of the shelter of the Sty and the self-explanation of an Air Force uniform. He expected that, like those children's party screamers which are all puffed out bravado until, blown to their paper extremity, they recoil hastily, gladly to the lips, some Pigs would need repeated puffs of confidence. Patently, at one period, among McIndoe's closest relationships with a former patient was that with Johnny Hills who remained many, many months at his home. A busy and public man spends much time between appointments and social engagements in the company of his chauffeur. Hills drove the Rolls.

Sorrowfully, one cannot now ask the surgeon if he knew Rudyard Kipling's story, 'The Tender Achilles'* and if that story had inspired his recruitment of Johnny Hills, but one can surmise! Kipling tells of two surgeons who are exchanging anecdotes. One surgeon, recalling a wartime operation upon a soldier, tells another that when the soldier was convalescent he was approached by him with an offer to become his chauffeur. But only he, the surgeon, knew that he had removed one-third of the man's brain!

Corporal Hills – and let it be established that he did not undergo brain surgery – had been working in a hangar when a bomber crashed into it and the petrol tanks exploded. His broken and burned body was recovered from the wreckage. Ground crew, he was ordinarily ineligible for membership of the club, but no true Guinea Pig could contemplate Johnny without the utmost compassion. Beyond his injuries, and few Guinea Pigs know this, there was as it happened an even more compelling reason why Johnny needed the club. Lying for weeks in his hospital bed he had had the time to wonder where he could find the answers to two questions which, in his physical distress, were large and frightening.

Who was he? Where was he born? Johnny Hills had never known.

Turning detective, Russell Davies brought peace to Johnny's mind. His mother had died during his father's war with the Germans, and his father had not come home. But, as Russell discovered, Johnny had a twin sister and Corporal Hills was thus enabled to look forward to a civilian future with an equanimity that might have eluded him for ever.

Johnny Hills had been in private service before the war and, as his strength returned, he began to consider the prospect of a new life abroad. His mother dead, his father disappeared, but his antecedents established, he sought the club's assistance in meeting this new ambition. At the Sty he had met Geoff Page's father-in-law, Nigel Bruce – Basil Rathbone's fruity Dr Watson in the pre-war Sherlock Holmes films. The Boss had admitted the film actor for an operation on an old wound of the first war. Now McIndoe, with Bruce's support, wrote to the British Consul-

*Limits and Renewals: Macmillan.

63

General in Los Angeles commending Johnny as a butler, preferably within the Hollywood community.

Alternatively Johnny enquired on his own account about emigration to Australia. The club assisted and he went. He worked very hard and built up a window-cleaning and lawn-mowing 'round' at Adelaide where he prospered as a man working for himself.

One day Blackie and Russell were discussing Guinea Pig business at Blackie's home. The conversation was interrupted by the arrival of a postman with a letter from Johnny Hills. He wrote of his children, David, two, Ann, four, Peter, six, and of the thirteen year old boy he had just adopted *to save him from having to grow up in an institution*. Johnny wrote also of his 'local' club member, Jack Wishart – 'Jack has been worried and it crossed my mind that, maybe, the club can help him.' Johnny explained that Jack now had three children and that, his old leg wound having broken down, his wife was working in a store. Jack, he said, would never dream of asking but could not his 40 per cent disability pension be reviewed in these circumstances?

Blackie handed the letter to Russell. 'Yours,' he said. 'Can do?'
'Sure.'

In the content of Johnny's letter from Australia, in that brief colloquial exchange at Barnstaple, there rested a blessing on the beliefs of the Boss and a guarantee for the future of the Guinea Pig Club.

\* \* \*

Although the Boss, Blackie and Russell have been the most leaned upon stanchions of the club, one would project an unbalanced picture were one not to include some of those others who, while not in such close and regular touch with so many Pigs, were glad also to carry their wartime connection forward to the present day. They, too, had been close enough to the Pigs in all their stages of recovery to understand the especial symptoms of social disability – how the uncertainties tumble over and over in the mind, surging, tossing like ragged bunting in some lunatic launderette; how social disability enlarges the bunting into flags the size of those Union Jacks which drape the bodies at a naval funeral, but never slip into the sea.

Some of the Pigs gravitated to these other friends, to surgeons Jerry Moore and Percy Jayes. To Connie McIndoe and to Elaine

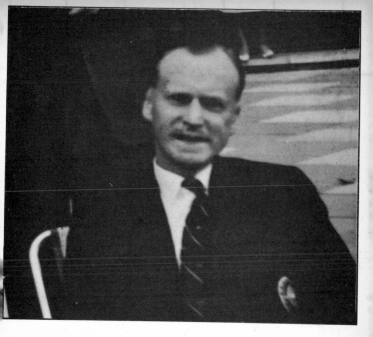

Sid McQuillan, a colliery clerk from Yorkshire, became a Guinea Pig after he emerged from the burnt-out nose of a bomber.

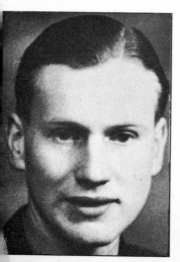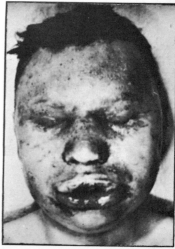

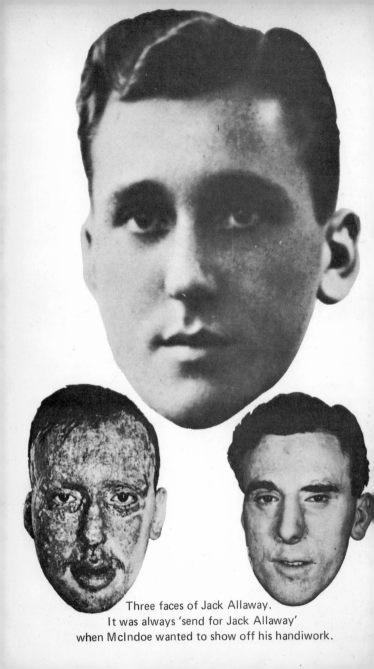

Three faces of Jack Allaway.
It was always 'send for Jack Allaway'
when McIndoe wanted to show off his handiwork.

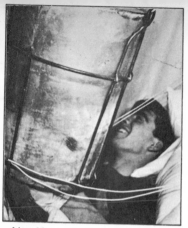
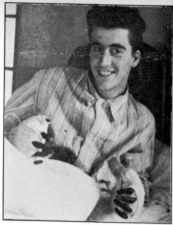

Alan Morgan's fingers were frostbitten over Leipzig. An attempt to save them in ice buckets failed, but in spite of this he became a jig borer controlling workings to a fraction of an inch.

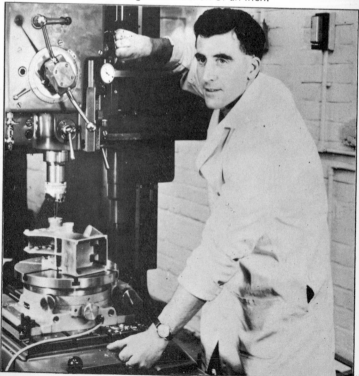

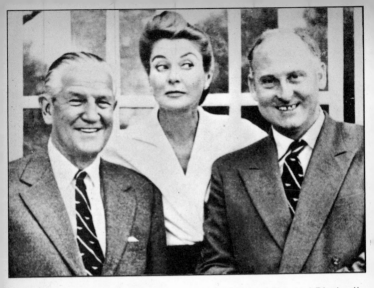

*Above:* Archie and Connie McIndoe with 'Blackie' Edward Blacksell.
*Below left:* Matron Hall pictured at the 1962 East Grinstead reunion.
*Below right:* A sense of humour was always encouraged.

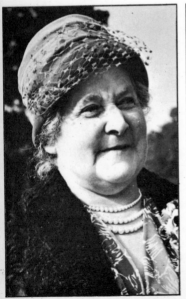

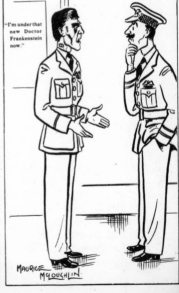

Blond, who, with her husband Neville, paid substantially to establish the McIndoe Memorial Research Unit at the Sty. To Elise and Douglas Stern of Felbridge whose hospitality has been prodigious.

Had it not been for the war and the chance which brought 'McIndoe's Army' to East Grinstead, comfortable, wealthy people like the Sterns would not have known and sometimes come to love such little people as the little man from Manchester who was to lean upon them. In the Sterns' England there were the rich, the better off, the acceptably off and the poor.

Excepting the doers-of-good-works most of those of any means did not mingle with those who could count themselves lucky if they received a weekly wage packet, and in no part of England were the taboos and distinctions so wide and apparent as in the homes and gardens which the wealthy had built among the salubrious pinewoods along the Surrey and Sussex borders; where servant girls from the depressed industrial north still staffed a household for a few shillings a week and their keep.

Like Johnny Hills, the man the Sterns befriended was another Guinea Pig who could not even offer the glamour of being air-crew. He was a square little man from Manchester, indistinguishable from thousands of other square little north countrymen who helped England without very much to thank her for, other than that, as Gilbert and Sullivan so eloquently remind us, he might have been 'a Roosian, a French or Turk, or Proosian, or perhaps Ital-ian'! Indistinguishable, that was, until the Air Ministry gave little George Hindley a balloon to care for, presenting a scene with all the pathos of a Stanley Holloway monologue.

They were winding in the balloon and he was guiding the great heavy cable which swung from it like a giant lead from a rogue elephant when it carried into a high tension cable, and Blackie remembers that when they brought Little George to East Grinstead Archie took one look at him and said 'he ought to be dead'. He was terribly burned and across the top of his head there ran a cleft, deep like a railway cutting in the Pennines and burned to more than the thickness of the cable. Little George Hindley was no longer indistinguishable from thousands of other north countrymen. Annually, a distinguished and distinguishable Guinea Pig, he attended the Guinea Pig weekend at East Grinstead where, with Group Captain Tom Gleave, the Chief Guinea Pig, he was a fellow guest of the Sterns. At the 1955 dinner, the Boss said: 'The impressive line of expensive cars parked outside indicates that the club has a number of prosperous members. The number of chaps who roll up in Jaguars at Guinea Pig dinners is encouraging.'

Little George also had a car although it was not a Jaguar. The Guinea Pig Club helped him to buy it so that he could continue to reach his work as a watchman, until ill-health enforced his retirement.

* * *

A pause for one reflection. The club's debt to Archie's, Russell's and Blackie's consistent involvement will now be clear. But these three men would wish it explained that the benefit of association has not been one-sided.

The surgeon's fashionable cosmetic practice thrived after the war in the sun of the unique personal publicity which the nature of the Guinea Pig Club made permissible.

If Russell Davies, with his selfless approach to medicine, deliberately and correctly has avoided any opportunity for financial gain or personal publicity, he has been rewarded by an ever increasing professional esteem at home and abroad.

Of the three men, however, it is East Grinstead's influence upon Blackie which has been the more fascinating. Guinea piggery, with its McIndoe-made contacts, was to create an opportunity from which he could orbit the world of entertainment, education, re-settlement and rehabilitation with the ideas which flood his brain – and yet remain headmaster of the Secondary Modern School at Barnstaple, and true to his vocation.

Bill Bourn, a Guinea Pig who like John Banham was a brewer, could not have appreciated how apposite was his comment when writing in another context from the brewery at Ndola on the borders of Northern Rhodesia, he said, 'Frankly, I formed the opinion that the patients were rehabilitating the staff!'

* * *

All the fingers of Alan Morgan – he will be remembered from Chapter three – were black and leathery. Horrible. When Ella, who was his girl friend from Manchester and who became his wife and the mother of their two boys, visited Alan, the black fingers stuck out uglily, frighteningly from the white bandages. 'Like dried bananas' Ella said. Alan was a skilled man whose skill depended greatly on the mobility of his hands. He need not have worn uniform because, as a jig-borer and a young man who had served an apprenticeship, he was in a reserved occupation. He discovered just how much of a key man his country considered him when he volunteered for the Navy and learned that he was not allowed to join. Disappointed he waited until, consequent upon the losses among bomber crews, his opportunity came as a volunteer for aircrew. The Royal Air Force gladly accepted such a skilled man and converted him into a flight engineer on 'Lancs'. On his 13th trip, and on the eve of his twenty-first birthday Alan, somewhat originally, earned his Guinea Pig brevet through frost rather than fire.

At 21, a lifetime as a civilian ahead, the sight of those useless fingers launched deep fears in Alan's mind. His skill and the living he could earn through it, depended on his hands and, as he or anybody else would have supposed, it would not be impossible for him to return to industry.

It worried Ella too, though she did not let Alan realise this, and Alan's natural anxiety increased when he learned that despite all efforts at the Queen Victoria hospital, his fingers would have to come off. There had always been hope while they were still there but the day came when the Maestro had to tell him that they were for 'the chop', the saddest aspect being that in McIndoe's opinion, had Alan received the correct treatment for frostbite at the hospital to which he was rushed after the Lancaster's emergency landing on the south coast, his fingers would have been saved.

Ella visited Alan frequently, making many journeys from Manchester to East Grinstead and on one trip she brought her fourteen year old sister. 'Whatever you do,' she told her, 'don't stare at any of the Guinea Pigs. Don't make them think you see anything peculiar about them.' At the same time, however, Ella often reminded Alan of how fortunate he was compared with most of his friends in the ward, some of whom had lost their faces and all or part of their eyesight.

Alan possessed another advantage over many of his fellow Guinea Pigs. Ella knew this but it was one point she did not, of course, stress with him. He had a steady girl friend whom he would soon marry. With a wife, she believed, Alan would make a better and more solid return to civilian life than some of the wild, unmarried men who formed the hard core of the gigantic 'boozing' parties which Ella soon appreciated provided the release for so many fears and inhibitions. What she did not know all those years ago was that however re-assuringly she could help Alan to return to civilian life, in those crisis moments which strain any man, Alan's experience and disability could, in certain circumstances, impose strain beyond his mental toleration.

Alan's crisis moment came when the company with which he had been employed throughout his civilian life was 'taken over' and he found himself without work.

Those who have been fortunate enough not to suffer disablement seldom appreciate how much it means to a disabled man to be accepted as a fully-functioning member of the community; to be able to 'work with his hands' however grotesque the antics of his stumps may appear to the uninitiated as they dart and prod and push, all the quicker for their need of speedier manoeuvrability, and on account of this, correspondingly monstrous in appearance.

When Alan had returned to his firm he convinced them that he could not only function fully as a jig-borer but also as a very good jig-borer. For months after his surgical operations he had practised and practised with what remained to him of one thumb on one hand, half a thumb on the other, but no fingers at all. He had started by wearing out pencil after pencil to write his name over and over again until he was sick of the sight of it and would have gladly changed his name. Apart from his thumb-and-a-half, the only help he had were the shallow clefts Archie McIndoe and his sugeons contrived for him, as they had for J.D. in order to help him realise his hospital ambition of seeing great trees crash down to his axe.

Indeed, Alan had trained himself with such determination that he believed, given a chance to persuade a medical board, he could return to aircrew service for long enough to gain his promotion from Sergeant to Flight Sergeant before demobilisation.

Alan told the Maestro; 'I'd like another bash in the air before it's too late.' McIndoe said: 'O.K., providing you can sell your hands to the Air Ministry.'

Alan did, and before his demobilisation, flew between Britain and Gibraltar as a Flight Engineer.

Back in civilian life, Alan's old firm knew of his skill, his mates knew him as a man, and his sense of security and of satisfaction in achieving his own very high standard of work as he went to the factory year after year had helped him to settle contentedly into a peacetime routine. Moreover, Ella had established a general store and at the time of rationing she managed to keep it healthily stocked with the help of explanatory letters written to suppliers by the Guinea Pig Club. In time, in fact, Alan became so convincingly re-established at his work that Ella, with two children to look after, felt safe in selling the shop in order to devote herself to her children, her home, and her husband.

But the men who manipulate money in the City of London, many miles and a world away from the muck where much of it is made, are not always knowledgeable about the individual heartbreak which their 'take-over' transactions can produce in a little industrial street. On the pristine foolscap laid place by place along the Board Room table, the figures announcing compensation to be paid with the final week's wages will appear generous to them. They will take a firm over and congratulate themselves upon their enlightened generosity. And go home to Surrey, Sussex, perhaps to East Grinstead where they may possibly number among the friends of the Guinea Pigs. But what they may not understand will be the hurt they unconsciously have done to a man like Alan Morgan. But it will not spoil their weekend because they will never have heard of the Alan Morgans of industrial Britain; of the men who were mutilated while many firms were making money out of the equipment with which Britain armed the men who became Guinea Pigs to save the nation from the terrors of German occupation.

Alan Morgan was given fair notice of his approaching 'take-over' dismissal but the 'sack' was followed by a serious nervous breakdown when he found that prospective new employers were pleasant enough at each interview – until they saw his hands. They could not believe that his skill was not only unimpaired, but enhanced by his determination to show himself more proficient than other men. They would not trouble to put his protestations to the test. Moreover, Alan states, his old firm refused to give him so much as a reference on their headed note-paper. Had Archie McIndoe been alive and had he heard of Alan's experience there would have been a river of managerial blood flowing through Manchester!

As it was Alan, perhaps foolishly, stubbornly harboured his distress to himself. But he did not appreciate the pressure the club is prepared to bring in such cases. He went downhill and by the time the club realised something was amiss, he was too ill to bother to explain his problem.

Alan Morgan's experience illuminates the one inevitable and

major disadvantage of the Guinea Pig Club's loose-knit organisation which depends upon the as-and-when, and often intuitive, attention of men who are wholly engaged in the new lives they have fashioned for themselves since their wartime and whole-time association with the Pigs.

Neither Alan nor Ella understood how forcefully the club would tackle prospective employers and on the other side the club was not wholly aware of Alan's problem. One hopes that this example will remind other members of the club to keep in touch with Blackie and Russell – the men who can help if and when they know *all* the story. Initiative from Pigs in difficulty is especially necessary because Blackie is a very busy headmaster and Russell is still 'passing them out'.

However, Alan Morgan's story ends happily, more happily than that of his former hospital friend, J.D. He recovered magnificently and there is no question that his great fortune in finding a company where managerial relations with the factory floor were of the very highest order, contributed. But is it not condemning of industry that having lost his work through no fault of his own, such a conscientious man should have to endure so much tribulation before being permitted an opportunity to prove that he had overcome his blatant disability?

\*       \*       \*

If ever a disabled airman could have paraded what remained of his hands in front of a medical board and finished with the dangers of wartime flying it was Alan Morgan, but he was not alone among Guinea Pigs in seeking, as he put it, 'another bash'.

Geoff Page, Frankie Truhlar, and a Canadian, Gordon Fredericks, number among Pigs who were repaired, returned to fight the enemy, and then, Oliver Twists of the club, came back to the Sty for 'more'. Richard Hillary's tragic story has been told too often, and too well by himself,\* to be related again here. But Hillary wrote one hitherto undiscovered and unpublished letter shortly before his death on a night-flying course, which throws new light upon the tragedy and reveals something of his state of mind when he returned to flying. The letter was written to the late Miss Wagg, sister of Alfred Wagg, first treasurer of the club, from the Officers' mess, R.A.F. Station, Charter Hall, near Duns, Berwickshire. It said: 'Dear Miss Wagg, I am here

\**The Last Enemy:* Macmillan

for three months "hard", learning to be a night fighter. When I say "hard" I mean it, not only the camp which is understandable, but also the effort of re-orientating oneself to two years ago. Still, I'm glad I've made the decision. I'm happier for it – as long as I can do the job. I'm finding this night stuff devilishly difficult.'

Throughout the war the Maestro found himself under heavier pressure than he would have wished from Pigs whose optimism paid little respect to their wounds. Among the most persistent must be counted Pilot-Officer William Dewar, of whom McIndoe informed a Medical Board: 'I have done no further work on this patient as he is very anxious to get back into action.'

When a German cannon shell had shattered Dewar's fighter cockpit over northern Europe in 1942, the thumb fell away from his right hand; the pilot received many other injuries and lost most of the sight in his left eye. That thumb was the second right-handed thumb in his life. It was a dummy thumb and had been fitted by McIndoe in the course of earlier surgery so that he could continue to control an operational aircraft.

By March 1943, Dewar had healed well and wore yet another new thumb, but his left eye was almost useless. The Maestro's memorandum continued: 'By the way, I would welcome some lead from you as to the disposal of one-eyed aircrew. I have a considerable number of them in my hands at the moment, all of whom are nagging away about flying. I would like, for instance, your views on (a) one-eyed pilots, (b) one-eyed radio-operators, (c) one-eyed air-gunners. However, I thoroughly recommend this one-eyed pilot to you.'

He could truthfully tell the Pigs he was doing his best.

There was one one-eyed Guinea Pig who flew several times before his defect was discovered. No names, no red faces!

Here it should be made plain that McIndoe's collaboration with patients anxious to return to operational service was not activated solely by a desire to please them. There were other factors. Firstly, early in the war, while there was a shortage of operationally trained and experienced airmen, it was his duty. Secondly, some Guinea Pigs – badly 'fried' though they may have been – were un-maimed and boisterously fit between surgical operations, fit enough to fight again. Thirdly, and this is the consideration which was of the most vital importance to the future welfare of members of the Guinea Pig Club, there were patients who patently would never fly again and would provide easy fodder for the invaliding boards. The more airmen McIndoe could return to squadron service the better the case he was building for the Long Term Treatment Scheme which he plugged and plugged to save other Pigs from being deprived of their Service status, uniform, pay, and even prospects, for some Pigs obtained promotion at the Sty.

The Long Term Treatment Scheme was, therefore, perhaps the most important concession won from Whitehall for the Guinea Pigs. McIndoe had been appalled by the official attitude that the sooner men whose hospital care was likely to exceed six months were invalided and pensioned, the tidier and the cheaper it would be.

Towards the end of the war when, following the personal intervention of Portal, Chief of the Air Staff, the long term scheme was working friendlily, and when trained operational aircrew were in fuller supply, the rate of repair and return began to decrease. It was a slowing-up process which was partly influenced by the state of the war, and partly by knowledge gained at the Sty, that some patients would appear to be able to tolerate only so many operations in a certain period and would then require a rest.

By the beginning of 1945, the year of victory in Europe and the Far East, even the spirit of guinea piggery was losing a little of its impetus. People everywhere were beginning to think about 'after the war'. This attitude invaded the Sty and one finds the Maestro recommending, as for Pig J. A. Sandeman-Allen, 'His treatment is now completed, but I do think that this young man has had enough and hope that you will agree with me that he should be invalided out of the Service'.

Nobody could dispute the assessment. This Flying Officer had been concussed in two serious crashes, wounded fighting over Singapore, and shattered by a shell which entered the cockpit of his Typhoon over France.

And there was this understanding note to the medical board in 1944 about another Guinea Pig whom it would not be fair to name:

'This Flying-Officer was badly burned over Berlin and the machine was brought home with very great difficulty, the result being the survivors of the crew were all decorated.

'Unfortunately the boy went absolutely cold on flying and remained so during his whole period in hospital. He has 25 operational flights to his credit, but has really developed the jitters.'

72

# CHAPTER SIX

'You may not yourself have bought it badly, but there are many who have and it is for these less fortunate Guinea Pigs whose will to live is as strong as ever that this Club really exists.'

The 'old' Reg Hyde, the young Reg Hyde who, before Germany invaded Poland went from Poole Grammar School into local government accountancy, ends where the strong growing dark and curly hair meets the new Reg Hyde along the plimsoll line of his plastic surgery, high on the forehead. The old Reg begins again somewhere beneath the new chin which Jerry Moore suggested in the course of the bomber navigator's seventy major surgical operations.

His nose, his eyelids, his face, much of his neck have been re-fashioned from skin grafted, or raised by pedicles, from the few parts of his body which escaped the flames when both engines of the Wellington bomber, in which he was instructing, cut, and Sergeant George Lamb who lost his life in the fire, put her nose down and crash-landed the 'Wimpy'.

Reg's hands were badly burned too and when one looks at the buckled fingers which proffer a tankard or manoeuvre the steering-wheel of his car, or help Jean Hyde pod the peas grown in their Crawley garden, one marvels at the will with which Reg, ten years behind his competitors, re-settled himself in civilian life as a qualified municipal engineer, passing his exams with but one concession gained on his behalf by the Guinea Pig Club – extra time to complete his papers because of the difficulty he experienced in writing and drawing.

Reg Hyde wears a blue blazer during the weekend and on the pocket is the badge of No. 49 Squadron, the Lancaster bomber squadron with which he had completed a tour of 'ops' over Germany before being posted to an operational training unit as an instructor. For a rest.

On the night of Reg's last flight the Wellington was returning to Silverstone from a cross-country training flight. There was a pupil crew of five with three instructors. Reg had put away his navigation instruments and was waiting for touch-down, thinking, 'Well, there's another night's work finished'. He stood up with his head in the Wimpy's distinctive astrodome to take a look round as the pilot made his approach. George Lamb, he thought, was making some comment over the intercom about the state of the starboard engine but Reg paid little attention to this as there had been heavy 'static' throughout the trip, and straining to understand the intercom had grown pretty wearying. Anyway, it was the end of the trip.

But then something happened which made him move very, very fast in the confined navigator's cabin. The port engine threw out a shower of sparks – and stopped.

'This,' Reg said, 'was where drill comes in. Automatically I thought – 'Crash-landing positions' and I took mine up by the main spar, feet up, facing the rear, and bracing myself with my arms.

'We were over the runway and I thought if we're lucky we'll get a jolt and everything will be O.K.'

But the trouble had developed at a decisive moment. Another aircraft was on the runway and normally Reg's pilot would have increased power and made a fresh circuit. The port engine gone and the starboard engine, as Reg remembers 'ropey', this was impossible. The only action the pilot could take was to put the nose down, overshoot the runway and attempt a crash belly landing. This he did, passing over the other aircraft which had landed safely, and in which Reg would have been instructing that very night had he not made a friendly swop in order to let another navigator, Eddie Warmington, take the ride because he had crewed with that pilot earlier in the war at Malta.

Many of the Guinea Pigs might have been less severely burned had they been wearing gloves or helmets and Archie McIndoe invariably asked them why they had not worn the protection provided by the Service.

Reg Hyde, who with Paul Hart and Godfrey Edmonds, number among the more disfigured members of the club, says: 'One never thought about catching fire. It seemed very remote. I never wore gloves as a navigator because I couldn't do navigational work in them and they weren't necessary in heated cabins, and I had whipped off my helmet thinking of the danger of getting trapped by an intercom lead tangled in the wreckage.'

Thus Reg braced himself in his crash position, gloves off,

helmet off and not contemplating the possibility of fire. But the Wellington's wings slapped into two trees and, as Reg described it, he found himself 'in the middle of a blazing bonfire'.

Feverishly, before taking up his crash position, Reg had tried to loosen the four bolts which held the astrodome, realising that almost certainly this would be his sole escape. He had loosened two bolts before the crash but after the impact he found that the astrodome had jammed. Struggling, he found himself growing more and more feeble. 'I thought I'd just about had it when the dome moved, and then the most extraordinary thing happened. One sometimes hears of people who discover superhuman strength in a moment of crisis. I would have found it difficult enough to escape through that hole in my fittest condition and yet I shot through there like a P.T. Instructor, although I had to pull myself up through a hole which was shoulder high.'

The fire was so intense that Reg could not see. He jumped on to the stub of one of the wings, both of which had been torn off by the trees and found himself up to the knees in the criss-cross geodetic construction which was a feature of the Wellington bomber.

The wing, like the rest of the aircraft, was well alight. He picked himself out of the wing and gave a shout. 'There was no reply, and after the roaring flames the silence seemed uncanny,' Reg recalls.

'I knew I had to get away from the wreck before it blew up. I climbed through a barbed-wire fence and over a ditch. It seemed so quiet. Just the steady crackling of the bomber and sheep bleating in the field.'

Reg learned later that there had been one other survivor. Upon impact, the rear-gunner was thrown clear and knocked unconscious. He was soon mended. He had merely broken an ankle.

Reg says that ignorance about burns saved many Guinea Pigs much mental torture. 'I simply didn't realise what had happened to me. I realised, of course, that I had been burned but I thought about burns in terms of scalding a hand with a boiling kettle, or of an accident with a hot iron, or even with a candle. When the ambulance delivered me at the R.A.F. Hospital, Halton, in October 1943, I thought "I'll stay here long enough to get some good Christmas leave, and then the treatment will be all over." I stayed there until May the next year, and even then, because the fire had burned away all the muscles, I could hardly open my mouth. I had to be fed and to drink through a rubber tube.'

When Archie McIndoe, on one of his rounds of what Pigs called 'the burneries' - the R.A.F. hospitals with burns units - suggested Reg's transfer to East Grinstead, Reg was pleased to leave. 'You get a bit hospital-bound and need a change of scene. Moreover there had been a recent hospital film show which featured the story of a beautiful girl who had suffered terrible facial injuries in a car crash and in the film she was made as beautiful as ever by plastic surgery. This gave me a lot of hope - false hope as it turned out - but it made me very keen to get to East Grinstead.'

By this time Reg's morale was very low. Far from being out of hospital by Christmas, it was now the beginning of the next summer and still he could not eat or drink. At the Sty they understood the importance of a patient's state of mind and when Jerry Moore said: 'We'll do your mouth so that you can eat', the surgeon knew that the hope of being able to eat and drink with the rest of the Pigs would raise Reg Hyde's spirits. For, without a mouth to control his food and drink, Reg had to lie flat on his back to take in any nourishment. Even so, three more years were to pass before Reg could drink without a rubber tube.

Jean and Reg Hyde have three handsome children, Susan, John and Peter. Some people in Crawley have remarked to Jean on the good looks and clear skin of her children and when this has happened Jean has known that behind the remark there has lain two unspoken questions - how can such a disfigured man be the father of such fine children, and was it right to take the risk of having them? It is only later, of course, when such people have stopped to think that they have realised that Reg's disfigurement is not congenital and that he cannot possibly pass it on.

The R.A.F. issued Reg with an 'escape' photograph of himself for use on forged identity papers in the event of coming down over Europe and attempting to escape with the help of the 'underground'. It is Reg's link with his true identity, and because he is still the same man within, it is how he feels himself to be, and the image in which his children are growing up. But comparison of the new and the old Reg makes the unthinking error of Jean's unthinking acquaintances understandable.

Jean says she never notices the disfigurement of any of the Guinea Pigs but she admits that this was not always so. She had taken a course in tropical nursing at the Hospital for Tropical Diseases before applying for a job at East Grinstead. 'I thought I'd seen some pretty gruesome patients among the returned

76

Japanese prisoners-of-war,' she said. 'I knew very little about the work at East Grinstead but I was intrigued when I applied for the post that I was asked to send a photograph. It seemed an odd way to select nursing staff for a hospital.

'I was even more surprised when I got there because on my third day two French airmen asked me to a cocktail party in the ward, and I thought "what a queer hospital!" The first time I went to an operating theatre, J.D. was on the slab and I thought "Frankenstein has nothing on this!".'

Reg Hyde, like so many Pigs, was transferred from an R.A.F. 'burnery' to East Grinstead at the Maestro's personal request. But not every serviceman with the requisite wounds was fortunate enough to be rescued from the harsher realities of R.A.F. or other hospitals.

It is an unhappy reflection upon the red tape which entwined patients and staff in Service hospitals that the bright and breezy, free and easy reputation at East Grinstead should have appeared so remarkable to the badly injured men who so gratefully were transferred there. Sam Gallop remembers with horror the rigid discipline of an R.A.F. hospital where it seemed ludicrous, as a legless man, to be commanded to 'Lie to Attention' when there was so little of him left. No legs to stiffen as the parade ground bellow filled the ward. Not even a jaw to broaden a grin at such nonsense. Like Sam's legs, most of it had gone.

Sam's schoolboy son Nicholas seems set to carry forward into his generation the Gallop desire to perpetuate the spirit of guinea piggery. He initiated a 'Squeakers Page' for the grown-ups' Guinea Pig magazine. 'Our Club,' he wrote in his first issue, 'is called the Squeakers Club because a young Guinea Pig squeaks and because our fathers are Guinea Pigs.'

\* \* \*

Some airmen, tantalised by stories of wards washed down with beer, wheedled their way to East Grinstead, as had Smith-Barry, their primeval predecessor. One or two came along at the invitation of Guinea Pig friendships struck up in bars, like the Fleet Air Arm pilot who, upon bemoaning his fate to Jimmy Wright, was whisked off to the Sty, ostensibly to deliver one blind, if not blind drunk, D.F.C. to his hospital. André Browne, who after two operational 'tours' as a fighter pilot, had crashed in a twin-engine aircraft with which as a single-engine pilot he was unfamiliar, owed his admission to a Canadian airman. Knowing about the new Canadian wing at the Queen Victoria Hospital the Canadian airman pleaded to be removed there so that he might be operated upon by his compatriot, R.C.A.F. surgeon Ross Tilley. Listening, ears-cocked in the next bed, André suggested that it might do his morale good if he accompanied the Canadian 'just for the fresh air and the trip'. As the Canadian was being tucked up in his new bed at the Sty, and André was saying goodbye, the Maestro walked into the ward. 'You can stay too,' he said.

André Browne was delighted, although in the middle of that night he wondered whether he had made a mistake. The bed of a badly burned Canadian caught fire.

\* \* \*

Certain pigs, like Sam Gallop, were broken and crunched, not 'fried', and that original title of the grogging club, the Maxillonians, gives the clue to why some of them were admitted to the Queen Victoria Hospital. The maxilio-facial unit was equipped to mend smashed faces and in the records of some of the Pigs there occurs the ugly word 'Dishfaced'. John Kirby earning this description when one engine cut during take-off in which he was learning twin-engined night flying, and instead of rising into the darkness of blacked-out Britain, he went smack into a concrete pill-box and started his career as a Guinea Pig.

It is, as will shortly be observed, a career of exceptional interest to this story because John Kirby, putting his thoughts about East Grinstead into his own words, reveals the Sty as a new Pig found it only one month after the founding of the 'grogging club' in 1941.

# CHAPTER SEVEN

'It has always been my belief that whenever he could a Guinea Pig should fall into a woman's arms but not into her hands.'

Only men can be admitted into membership of the Guinea Pig Club, but the Sty was not, of course, an all-male world and it would be unchivalrous to carry the club's story further without recalling the devotion of Matron Hall and her nurses, many of whom, in company with Sister Meally of Ward III, became 'Mrs Pigs'.

It is a very exceptional woman who will accept prolonged disturbance of her ordinary domestic routine. Ponder then the nightmare situation of Matron Hall when war brought an unruly invasion of her tidy little cottage hospital at East Grinstead, led by a surgeon who rolled barrels of beer into her wards and whom patients and staff named 'the Boss'.

To Matron Hall and Sister Cherry Hall, her sister, who both later retired to Ireland, whence like so many Irish girls they came to nurse in England, the Guinea Pigs are in debt for more than good nursing. Without their co-operation and through them that of all the pre-war and wartime nursing staff, there might have been no club, and in some families, no Piglets like the three Hydes to carry on the East Grinstead tradition. Only a matron in a million would allow her hospital to be treated like a Grand Hotel, her night sisters like night porters to let in the revellers and set up the nightcaps and sandwiches, and her wards as wings of a Club House with a twenty-four hour licence.

Jimmy Wright and 'Flash' McConnell, returning from a London night club, walked into the ward at 5 a.m. one morning as the night sister was doing her last round. She had been there only a few days. 'Oh you are up early, are you going somewhere?' she asked.

André Browne remembers that on occasion the ragging became so violent that, in his opinion, some of the Pigs went too far and a nurse would leave a bedside in floods of tears. 'But,' says André, 'the Maestro would walk in and take the side of the Pig.

79

"These men have put up with the hell of a lot and so you can put up with just a little nonsense," he would tell nurses who went overboard.'

A fragment written shortly after the Battle of Britain by a fighter pilot who did not identify himself – it was found loosely among some pensions correspondence of Russell Davies – will assist understanding of Matron Hall's remarkable contribution towards encouraging just the correct amount of conspiracy between her staff and her patients.

This Guinea Pig had returned to the hospital. 'Two days late,' he wrote, 'to undergo the first of a long series of operations to make my face and hands a more presentable picture.

'The Matron greeted me and I hastily explained to her that the air-raids in London were the cause of my being two days late. An amused twinkle came into her eyes. It was quite obvious she knew that I had spent the last two days painting London a dark shade of red.'

Richard Hillary in 'The Last Enemy' has left a sophisticated impression of the hospital and a tribute to its nursing staff but later in the war there were some very different inhabitants of the beds. The Henry Standens, the Jack Topers, the George Hindleys, the Alan Morgans of the Guinea Pig Club. The men who came from the little back streets, clerks' stools, the drapers' shops, the government schools, to replenish the bomber crews as losses mounted over Berlin, Hamburg, Essen, Dusseldorf, Frankfurt – and many of the other places the airline pilots will take you to today. These men form the core of the Guinea Pig Club and were the men of whom their Maestro was thinking when he said, 'As we worked a persistent question nagged at my mind: When their bodies are whole again can we also rebuild something of their lives?'

John Kirby was one of these men. He was not so well educated as the early Battle of Britain pilots, but he could *feel* and what he felt he described. His picture of the Sty reflects, unintentionally, the nightmare of Matron Hall and how she and her nurses maintained hospital efficiency throughout all the high jinks; how they drummed on persistently while the Maestro and his Pigs blew the trumpets.

John Kirby writes:

'I was not fried and as a result I was shunted into Ward I. I had never been a patient in a hospital before although I had been a visitor on several occasions. When I looked round Ward I, I

80

began to wonder. I must say that, except for the beds with 'bods' in various stages of repair, I thought that it would make a good barrack block or storehouse. The beds were forces' issue. Low black things with spring mattress. Strangely enough I was not upset by this impression. There just seemed to be an atmosphere of efficiency.

'After the hospital beds of Innsworth (where he had been taken initially), I felt that I was much too near the floor. Doctors and nurses seemed to be looking down from a great height.

'I arrived at midday. The next morning someone came and pushed something like clay in my mouth. What the hell was going on?

'I soon found out. A set of splints were cemented to my jaws, both upper and lower. A carpenter came down the ward with long pieces of two-by-two and started to erect a scaffold over my bed.

'Up to this point I had no idea what was going on. I was so bemused. . . .

'These splints are giving me hell. They are not only encasing my teeth but also parts of my gums. A post is erected at the head of the bed and another at the foot with a connecting piece across the top. No fuss. No bother. Just Heath Robinson sort of material. The scaffold is ready. Where's the hangman?

'Here he comes. Funny he isn't wearing a mask. He has a round, kindly face and gives the impression that he knows what he is going to do. I remember I had seen him before when I first came into this "hospital".

'Round face was talking to his assistant about "middle third borkum beam", or that's what it sounded like. All double Dutch to me. Two pulleys were put on the cross beam and the Boss and his assistant – a brown job named Captain Sheffield – produced a piece of cord. This was attached to the hook on the top set of splints, over the pulleys and Lo! and Behold! bags of shot, or the like, were tied to the end. After another inspection the chief and his assistant left me.

'Here come the nurses and I think it must be Sister with them. Slim, unsmiling, severe. Oh so severe. "Take that pillow away." Glory be! she's Irish.

'When everything was shipshape they left me. I wish I knew what was going on. They had left me strung up like a stuck pig.

'My bloody ribs are aching like hell but I can't turn over. This damned cord keeps me flat out on my back. I suddenly realise that I have only one useful eye. The right eye doesn't seem to be open. It doesn't seem to matter.

'I remember vaguely seeing my wife when I was at Innsworth. Where is she now? After a few days my wife came in to see me and I was shocked. I have read novels in which the author describes a person's eyes as "dead". I suddenly realised what they were trying to convey. My wife's eyes had no expression. They were "dead". Yes, I was beginning to notice things, even with only one eye.

'Sister Harrington was still the same severe person. Everything must be just so. I wonder where she was trained.

'After about a fortnight I was beginning to waken up. Groups of R.A.F., Army, and Navy officers would occasionally gather round my bed and someone would give them a lecture. In this way I began to piece together what had happened and also what was being done to straighten me out.

'The upper jaw was gradually responding to the pressure of the weights and was coming out. Eventually the constant pressure pulled the jaw out but even now only two teeth meet. There was a gap of something like one eighth inch between my front teeth. Strong elastic was put on to hooks and down, oh so slowly, came the top set.

'The day came when my front teeth overlapped. The elastics came off and on went some wire fixed by a pair of pliers.

'Now I can get rid of these weights. These ribs have given me hell. After my mechanic has finished I ask the Captain to take off the cord. He walked to the end of the bed, lifted the weights, stood for about ten seconds, put the weights back again, then came and asked me if I had felt any pain. I'll say I had. It seems that the top jaw was trying to go back and I had, during those few seconds, a terrific pain just in front of my ears. No, it was going to be a gradual process.

'There is a Doctor Jayes keeps coming round and one day he sprang a surprise. (This was Mr Percy Jayes, the plastic surgeon, who later sprang another surprise on the Guinea Pigs by marrying the "severe" Sister Harrington.) "Do you drink beer or stout?" – Can a duck swim!

'When the shock wore off I found that I was to have half a pint of beer every day. Taffy and I shared a pint to the envious glances of the rest of the boys.

'Now that I was beginning to take stock I saw the aforementioned Taffy walking about with a tube from his face into his dressing gown. Jacky across the ward was taken down into the "block" at regular intervals. One day's peace. Then he was back to his usual chatty self.

'There is a wind rushing down the ward but I cannot see what is going on. The movement is working up the ward. Now I see the old beds are being replaced by pukka hospital beds. All, that is, with one exception. Mine!

'I still have my scaffold. My bed spoils the new look. The fellow in the next bed is beginning to revive and leans over to have a chat. We begin to get to know each other. John Bubb had returned from his first op with a broken jaw and smashed leg. Something about bullets in his turret.

'Lying there with only a limited field of vision, mainly the roof, I had plenty of time to think and listen. I recall that at Innsworth I was given the usual hospital rations. A square of cheese, a piece of marge, a piece of bread. I didn't eat any of the food. I couldn't.

'My wife used to bring custards and a sloppy food supplied by the kindly person who gave her a bed near the hospital.

'At this place I am on what they call jaw food. I am not the only one on this slop. There must be several of the boys in the same boat, judging by the number of feeding mugs that are on the tray.

'I am surprised at the way the hospital is run. Some of the fellows who are able to get out don't always come back after tea. After about 7.30 p.m. everybody seems to settle and all is peace and quiet until 10, 11 and even 12 p.m. Then I hear sounds of return of the merrymakers. I must still be delirious. That fellow is drunk. It would never happen in hospital. You can see I was still a new boy.

'The great day arrives. The man everyone referred to as Mac, the Boss, gave permission for the cord to be taken off. Glory be! I can turn on my side. All these weeks I have had to lie flat on my back whilst someone came and made my bed, gave me a bed bath, took the dressings off my hands, picked off the scabs, messed about with the cuts on my face. There was a nurse seemed to be an expert at these picking operations.

'Now I can turn and see my neighbours but even now I can't see right down the ward. I am still in the low bed. The next day I get the new bed. The ward is now completely re-equipped. I remember the pleased expressions on the faces of the doctors and sisters. Even Sister Harrington smiled and nodded with satisfaction and somehow I felt better. I had been the blot on the landscape, holding back the improvement and smartness. Now I was not a drawback. Don't misunderstand. No one had by glance, remark or in any way suggested that I was the odd man out. I just know.

'I now had visions of sitting up, let alone having a pillow but all that was squashed by Sister. "You can have one pillow." She said it in the same tone that I imagine Scrooge would use when giving away a crust. Although she was so unbending I had developed a great feeling of confidence in our Sister. She knew just what I could be allowed to do and although I sometimes tried to persuade her to let me sit up I was now prepared to accept her word. I'm afraid I pulled her leg, or rather I tried. She seemed so unbending. Two pillows then I was allowed as back rest just for a few minutes so that I could shave.

'The bloody ward is on a turntable. I can't keep my face in the mirror. I'm damned well not going to get down until I have shaved. At last I have had a scrape. What a relief to lie down again but don't let Sister know. She may not let me have it tomorrow. I didn't fool her for one minute.

'Here comes Robby with his plaster jacket and arm in the air. Last night he was allowed out to a dance. He and Jacky took my wife. They were both stinking when they came back and Robby lay on his bed incapable except for his voice. He proceeded to give a performance of barrack room songs. The nurses on night stint got these two undressed and put them to bed.

'I have never ceased to admire those girls, most of them V.A.D.s, coping with situations like that. The next time the boys went out they again took Ginger and the wife, and at about midnight there was a knock at the window against my bed. I opened it and took in the four bottles of "milk". This milk run became a regular operation and John Blubb and I used to have our own celebrations.

'There was a sailor on the opposite side of the ward. His mouth was always watering when I had my half pint ration. He got himself organised and had his regular supply of medicine.

'I had to laugh at his description of his first trip out. He was taken out in a chair which had pockets at the side and back. When the chair left the hospital it was loaded with empty bottles. When they got on to the drive there was such a rattling and clanking of bottles that they had to sing loud and long to hide the sound. Half way down the drive they met the Boss. . . .

'Came the day when the plaster is taken off my ankle. This is painful. The plaster is stuck to the hairs on my leg. Oh don't pull. It's surprising how comparatively small things seem much more painful. I was still one-eyed. My right eye is still closed but I am still "cocky". I tell the doctors that I know that I shall get better and that I shall go back flying. They shake their heads. Time goes by and I am allowed to get up. I am shocked when I am allowed to take my first bath. My legs are only about the same thickness as my arms. Gradually I improve and then I am told I can go into East Grinstead. Not alone. I must have a chaperone. My right eye is now open but the sight has not yet returned. I realise that everything is not quite as it should be. My guide saves me when I try to step down a double curb with one step. I'll have to go carefully.

'My teeth are freed from the wire and Mr Ridley, the eye specialist, invites me to a Rotary Club Lunch. The main course was fish. I remember how awkward I was with my knife and fork.

'My first night out. A Red Cross dance. Everyone is so kind. The people of East Grinstead are the most kindly and understanding people I know. There is one person I shall always remember, the late Mrs Fraser. A most charming person in every way.

'My stay at E.G. was filled with incidents. Like the night we got back to the annexe at 1 a.m. We tried the windows. None would open. Matron greeted us from the front entrance, inviting us to enter by the door.'

The Guinea Pigs' relationship and debt to Matron Hall and her nursing staff is implicit in John Kirby's simple, telling narrative. It will, therefore, surprise the uninitiated, that as has been stated previously, there are no women members of the club.

McIndoe wanted to open the door to them. At the annual meeting of the club in 1945 he sought a precedent by prevailing upon Flight-Lieutenant Harold Stannus, an Australian Pig, to move the immediate election of Sister Jill Mullins, McIndoe's theatre assistant, and of Sister Meally of Ward III. McIndoe supported the motion from the chair. It suffered a heavy defeat. Australian Pig George Taylor, recalls: 'The Boss accepted the decision with good grace and a democratic spirit, but it was the only time I can recollect a failure by him to sway a body of Pigs to his way of thinking.

'Probably there was not one person in the room who did not want each of those two wonderful girls to be one of us, but it was felt that the Guinea Pig Club was a men's club and ladies should join the Pigs as guests. Further, there were others to be considered – Matron Hall, Sisters Cherry Hall, Harrington, Polly Walker and Mary Rae.'

\* \* \*

Men fall in love with their nurses. Some marry them. Many do if they are Guinea Pigs, or as it sometimes seems, are associated with Guinea Pigs. The late Sir Victor Sassoon, who paid for one of the club's annual dinners out of St Paddy's Derby winnings and whose widow endowed the club with some of St Paddy's subsequent stud fees, married *his* nurse.

The patient-nurse marriage incidence at the Sty was high, and as so many men do not marry the women they *think* they love but find themselves married to the women who love them, many of the nurses fell in love with Pigs, the Pigs proposed and Britain is satisfactorily sprinkled with Guinea Piglets.

Other Guinea Pigs rooted beyond the Sty for their romance, finding love in some odd places. Gus Fowler, who had been a tea planter in Assam before the war, met his wife in a nudist camp.

Guinea Pig marriages have foundered, but not beyond the usual pattern. Men who were the most incapacitated have remained married. Cynics in the club say that is because you can't leave home when your legs are locked up in a cupboard for the night and the wife sleeps with the key under her pillow.

Nevertheless, McIndoe was reminded frequently that the ordinary pitfalls of marriage can become canyons for a Guinea Pig. Towards the end of the war and for a few years afterwards the club's matrimonial correspondence was heavy and Blackie, Russell and the Boss were taxed by such awkwardness as that of the Pig whose future wife was expecting before club-aided divorce proceedings had started. Or of the Pig who wrote: 'You may be able to recall our discussing my somewhat unhappy matrimonial problems when I was last at the hospital some two years ago having my left eye removed.'

Occasionally the President of the club unleashed himself on the subject of Guinea Pigs and marriage but when he did his words presented a remarkable blend of re-proof, humour, practical advice, irony and humanitarian understanding. At the annual dinner in 1950, he said:

'You will remember that the problems of Guinea Pigs during the five war years were really comparatively simple ones, though

86

they involved big principles. These, I used crudely to say, concerned women, jobs and money. They were solved by methods well known to you.

'The past five years have, however, brought to light many more complicated tangles in the field of human relations; the result of all the forces at work when you combine physical disability with marriage and with the struggle for survival in this anxious and uncertain world. When you ask us for help in this field we are often at our wits' end to know what to say or do – whether to advise or remain silent.

'It has always been my belief that, whenever he could, a Guinea Pig should fall into a woman's arms but not into her hands; that while it is important that, if possible, you should find and cleave to the one woman in the world who will make you supremely happy, it is much more important that you should avoid the thousands who can make your life supremely miserable. I do realise, of course, that this little bit of advice is somewhat late for you have mostly made your selections and are now reaping the benefits of the whirlwind.

'It is somewhat disquieting to note, however, that domestic problems are on the increase and, while we have done what we can, we do not profess to be very proficient in delivering Solomonic judgements – where the wife has decided that the handsome Romeo down the street is more desirable than her slightly singed Guinea Pig, or on the contrary, where the slightly singed Guinea Pig has decided that if he can't get the plums out of a cake he will feel better if he kicks the missus. Tolerance and understanding between two people will do more in this field than third-party interference and I commend this course to those of you who stand in need of it.'

Thus far would McIndoe go. He steered the Guinea Pig Club into many agencies, including a thriving, string-pulling employment agency, but there were two roles he was determined the club must not play. Those of marriage bureau and marriage guidance council.

For the first there was certainly no call. In 1952 one finds him replying to an offer of a job for an *unmarried* Guinea Pig schoolmaster which had reached him from the little West Indian Island of St Vincent:

'The trouble is there are few bachelors left, most of them having a wife and six starving kids. Those who have stayed single are certainly not in the field of education.'

# CHAPTER EIGHT

'We've had some mad Australians,
Some French, some Czechs, some Poles,
We've even had some Yankees,
God bless their precious souls.
While as for the Canadians –
Ah! That's a different thing,
They couldn't stand our accent
And built a separate wing.'
(*Last verse of the Guinea Pig anthem.*)

Blackie wrote the words of the Guinea Pig anthem. He says it was because he had become rather bored by the maudlin singing of 'The Church's One Foundation' in the Old Brown Cow, the Guinea Pigs ramshackle bus, returning to the Sty from so many drinking excursions. The anthem has lasted but the mood in which it is sung annually at the dinner has changed since the Old Brown Cow's riotous journeys.

Like their author, Blackie, eternally young and enthusiastic within, the words of the anthem have not changed. Only their emphasis. In the bus they were sung without much thought. A parochial alternative to 'She'll be Coming Round the Mountain', or perhaps to, 'Nellie Deane'. Now at the dinner when two hundred of the surviving members of McIndoe's army rise to sing them, Blackie's words which jestingly had been called an anthem, hold the quality of a hymn. It is a solemn interval on a jovial night. The men who sing are remembering with the intensity that one observes two minutes' silence on Armistice Day. The 'mad' Australians and the Canadians who built a separate wing, are the most warmly remembered.

Canadian airmen served in their own Royal Canadian Air Force squadrons and individually with the R.A.F. Fire does not differentiate. Canadian bodies burn as quickly and as badly as British or Australian or New Zealand. The men from these Dominions of the British Empire, as those nations were still proud to know themselves, had crossed thousands of miles of ocean to defend their mother country in her European struggle.

They did not know it then but they had also come to provide a future emotional background against which, as now it must seem to some of them and to their children, that Britain's attempted mercantile commitment to Europe, is an act of ingratitude. They had come in such numbers and with such zest, that soon they were in as much need of the Sty as the Maxillonians.

There were many more Canadian Pigs than Australians, New Zealanders or airmen from the other Empire countries. Canada is larger in population and was capable of training more airmen. As the Canadian casualties increased, it grew plain that the bursting Sty, this expanded cottage hospital, could not continue to offer them its especial facilities without swift and more solid building than the huts at the back.

Canada understood. She moved in her Royal Canadian Engineers. She provided her own materials. She built a large wing for the little hospital. She shipped her own doctors, surgeons and nursing sisters to East Grinstead and when Germany had been defeated, she shipped them all home to the Maritimes, the Prairies and the Rockies with equal speed and she presented her wing to the Queen Victoria Cottage Hospital of East Grinstead.

Canadians do not sentimentalise 'the old country' or life as readily as Australians or New Zealanders. Consequently, the Canadian Pigs have not kept a similarly close liaison with the club and with each other. The war in Europe ended, they bestowed upon the Maestro the ceremonial honour of hauling down their flag at the hospital and dispersed.

In contrast with the Australians, who, as will be explained shortly, were nature's Guinea Pigs, they never responded to the emotional appeal of guinea-piggery. Their outlook was practical. Like the purpose with which they built their wing, made a film there to prepare Canadian families for the return of their disfigured and crippled sons, and then left!

Individually the Canadian airmen also tended to be as practical. They were apt to be more opportunist than their fellow Pigs, some using the surgical, humanitarian and high level contact-making opportunities at East Grinstead with great benefit to themselves. The experience of Flight-Lieutenant Gordon Fredericks, a Canadian Observer who, eventually was to re-cross the Atlantic holding the double distinction of a bar to his Guinea Pig badge and a Cambridge degree, is an example.

Following a second set of injuries – his Mosquito returning from an operational sortie crashed into the sea – Fredericks was taken to an R.A.F. hospital where he found conditions anything but congenial after East Grinstead. He wrote to the Consultant Plastic Surgeon to the Royal Air Force, 'Dear Mac, Well, I've gone and done it again. It just came apart in me 'and sir. It's pretty hard to show a profit on me. I only hope it won't tie me up too long and cost me my chance to bag a Hun. The thing that has shaken me is landing in this concentration camp. I must say the place could do with a touch of your rationalising influence. It's quite a contrast to our beloved E.G. The strangest part to my way of thinking is how little the boys seem to know about what is wrong with them and what is being done about it'. This last sentiment is of especial note in the story of the club because it provides further evidence in support of the value of McIndoe's decision to risk the creation of an army of hospital bores discussed earlier.

In fact a remarkable change had been wrought in Fredericks since encountering McIndoe, the Guinea Pig spirit, and possibly the most important of all in his case, the Guinea Pig propensity for string-pulling. For here was an airman who, at the beginning of his first visit of seven months to East Grinstead had arrived so embittered that all he could think about was an early trip home to Canada. And now, after a second set of injuries, he was seeking a quick return to action.

Blackie, Russell and the Maestro had been asking themselves why Freddy, as they all knew him, was not running true to form. Normally, as they had learned from experience, the first reason why those who were anywhere near fit to fly wished to return to their squadrons, was the fear that others might think they were hiding behind their wounds. McIndoe employed this natural and understandable fear to help him to do his duty as he saw it while the war situation was critical and so long as the shortage of operationally trained airmen like Fredericks remained.

With Fredericks, however, during his first period at East Grinstead, it seemed that a different fear prevailed and after a while Freddy confided it to the Maestro. It was, that having almost completed one tour of operations in an obsolete aircraft, the torpedo-carrying Hampden, he was extremely apprehensive about flying again in the type of aircraft in which he had crashed. He told McIndoe that he felt it not unreasonable to request an aircraft in which he could place confidence and to be posted to a Command in which the circumstances of his first mishap would not be duplicated.

The surgeon took the point immediately and asked Fredericks to be specific. 'I would like to be posted to a Mosquito squadron', said the airman, 'and I would prefer bomber Mosquitos because I believe they give a little more scope to the Observer.'

A few days later McIndoe wrote personally on Freddy's behalf to 'Sammy' Hoare, the Mosquito intruder ace: 'My dear Hoare, I wonder if you would be good enough to see and talk with Flying-Officer Gordon Fredericks, R.C.A.F. He is a very experienced Observer who had the misfortune to crash in a Hampden seven months ago, sustaining fairly severe burns, from which he has now completely recovered. . . . His fancy seems to be in Mosquito work.'

Repaired a second time at East Grinstead, after his Mosquito mishap, the club 'organised' Freddy into Cambridge and helped him through a number of financial vicissitudes until the Boss was delighted to receive,

'Dear Archie. Have a drink on me and see that John and Russell get one too. I got a First. . . . My real thanks are to the Club which made it possible.'

McIndoe replied, 'My dear Freddie. A thousand congratulations on your results. It is simply magnificent and everybody here (the Sty) is pleased beyond words. I am sorry that you are off to Canada so soon but I am sure you must be looking forward to it. In any case it has all been worthwhile *and the Club feels honoured by your success.*'

* * *

Nobody said, 'Make Jack Allaway the star of a film, it is the only occupational therapy which will return him to people'. Not even Blackie. Where they believed it would work the Boss and Blackie indulged Pig fancies as those of pregnancy. However, even they, with all their resource and McIndoe's nourished connections in the world of entertainment, would have been exercised to arrange a starring role for Jack Allaway, who had lost much of his face in a bomber crash. Extraordinarily, the Canadian government brought Jack this unlikely opportunity.

Anticipating the repatriation of the first Canadian Guinea Pigs, there was official concern about their reception. Canada, therefore, authorised the shooting of a documentary film at East Grinstead – 'New Faces for Old'. When the film unit arrived at the hospital no Canadian Pig was advanced sufficiently in repair to take the starring role. Fortuitously, Jack Allaway, whose self-consciousness had been worrying Blackie and the Boss, stepped into the part. Sewing Canadian shoulder flashes and badges on to Jack's service tunic, a nurse converted the Birmingham sergeant into an 'acting' Canadian. Soon, by following Jack's career at the Sty, Canadians as distant as Medicine Hat were to learn how their boys were being cared for in a very English, if less convincingly named, place, East Grinstead.

Enthusiasm in any man is an enormous personal asset. In a Guinea Pig it is gold. To encounter prancing enthusiasm in a disfigured and maimed man, is to experience an uplift equivalent to a pint of Black Velvet on the morning after the night of the Guinea Pig dinner. Some Pigs were born dour and despite all the bonhomie of their East Grinstead days, such men remain dour Guinea Pigs. Theirs is the advantage when the outlook is bleak. They take the 'downs' the more easily. But meet a Pig who is an enthusiast and is 'up' and one is swept along with the tide race. Alan Morgan, whose 'down' temporarily destroyed him, became one of the great enthusiasts in the club. His enthusiasm for his jig-boring machine, his bouncing description of its infinite potentialities, his thanksgiving that with no fingers, half a thumb on one hand and a whole thumb on the other, he could work to 0.00015 inch on a jig-boring machine, had to be heard to be believed. Jack Allaway, describing the profitable sale of his first shop in Birmingham and how business prospects opened out for him at Crawley, is another great Guinea Pig enthusiast. But he had experienced his 'down' and not always had it been thus.

One learns this when Jack's eyes grow serious within the rings of pale, motionless skin with which plastic surgery repaired his face and as he feels contemplatively down his new nose, which was raised by pedicle from the skin of his chest and says quietly, 'One of the best Mac did, isn't it? But he was lucky with my grafts. Everything took. It was always "send for Jack Allaway" when Archie wanted to show his handiwork off'.

Jack was the wireless operator of a Hampden bomber. He had returned from a shipping strike in the Skagerrak when a Ju 88 intruder sneaked-up on the Hampden's tail and shot it down as it was about to land in Norfolk. 'We were making our approach when I saw the tracers. We caught fire and I thought "this is the end". When I realised I had survived the crash, I found I couldn't open the cupola above me. My hands were burned. I was not frightened. I thought of mother at home. I just thought I wonder what she's going to think when I've gone. Honestly, I was quite prepared to stay there and wait. I heard a scream. I suppose it was the navigator. Then I looked down and saw daylight. I dropped through the hole into a ditch and scrambled into a ploughed field. My hands had been badly burned because I'd taken my gloves off and was getting my gear together, thinking, well that's another one safely over – my twenty-fifth in fact.'

Jack was six months at the R.A.F. hospital, Ely, before removal to the Sty. 'Wing Commander George Morley did my temporary eyelids there and Archie McIndoe trimmed them up later.

'Towards the end of my time at Ely I grew pretty impatient. I wanted them to hurry up but with contraction from burns you can't hurry. You've got to wait, for instance, for your eyelids to finish their contraction. So there you are with whopping great eyelids and wondering whether you'll always look like that.

'I was so anxious', Jack says, 'that one day Archie brought along a chap who'd been through it before the war. "This is what you'll be like", he said, "but it will take time."

'See my nose. That's a very good nose, I reckon, but it took twelve months. There it was like a lump of plasticine to begin with. Archie had to sculpture it, take the fat away, put in the nostrils.'

In common with his fellow Guinea Pigs and most people, Jack Allaway had never considered what burning does to a body. It was something aircrew did not begin to think about. The degree of some of the Guinea Pigs' burns is evidence of the distressing result of a failure to rationalise between acceptance of the danger of fire and the encumbrance of protective gloves, helmets and goggles. Tom Gleave's goggles were up but he was wearing his favourite gloves 'a thin, pansy unofficial type' he says. Even with this protection his fingertips were so burned that, by removing his fingerprints, the enemy provided him with a passport to undetectable burglary had he wished to resort to crime! Nevertheless, his hands were only slightly crippled. Jack Mann's goggles were up when, eyes tight shut, he crash-landed his blazing Spitfire . . . Jack Allaway had taken his gloves off and was putting his gear away. . . . The evidence repeats and repeats itself.

If, however, this refusal to accept the possibility of severe burning and lack of appreciation of the effects of burning lead in many cases to injuries, the degree of which might sometimes have been lessened, correspondingly it reduced awareness as the

Pigs lay in hospital of the ravages of the fire which had consumed them.

'You don't realise for quite a while that you are going to look different', Jack Allaway says. 'If you have ever seen a burned man before, you wonder, "what's happened to him" and you tend to think that perhaps he was born like it.' This, Jack believes, helps to explain why so many people are so surprised, initially, when they meet Guinea Pigs who are happily married and have children who are among the most handsome in the land.

'It's when you get a bit better', Jack remembers, 'that you begin to think, "well, perhaps I *do* look a bit different". It was at Ely where, unlike East Grinstead, there was not a ward full of other Guinea Pigs to help you get used to the idea, that I caught the reflection of myself in Sister's office window from twenty feet away. I was too scared to go any closer and I turned away quickly. I thought, "you look like a chimpanzee". That was because I was looking straight at my nostrils.

'At first when I was well enough to go to the toilet I couldn't bring myself to look in the mirror. Then I took a quick peep, a very quick peep. I thought, "It's just not you. It's like looking at somebody else". I was too scared to take a second look.

'Next time I was a bit more daring. I took a closer look and looked just a little longer. It was very odd. I felt the same person and yet it just wasn't me.

'Can you imagine? You know what you look like. You go to a mirror and you see someone quite different. And, just as strange, your fingers are locked in one position and yet they feel the same as they were before being burned.

'Slowly you come to accept it. Then you begin to say, "Well, I'm not too bad." Then you find the courage to really study yourself at different angles and when you get to East Grinstead where there are so many others, you find yourself saying "And I'm certainly not as bad as poor old so and so."

'And very soon, when you begin to get out and about you make your greatest discovery. You find that girls don't go for good looks. The good looking fellow can't just click his fingers and they all come running. They don't.'

With some Pigs it was much to the contrary. Letters were received at the Sty from women who preferred disfigured men – not for their great hearts but from a perverse attraction for their scars and weals. When a particular Pig was specified the patient was asked discreetly to what extent he was interested in the woman – if he knew her. If the Pig desired no further contact she was brushed firmly off!

Later, after the film which the Canadians made, had helped to restore Jack's confidence, Billy Butlin stepped in with an offer which was to contribute to the increase of confidence among a number of Guinea Pigs. He offered them jobs at his holiday camps. At the Clacton camp Jack met Joan who, following demobilisation from the A.T.S., was working there as a waitress. They married and had piglets.

\*　　\*　　\*

One has eulogised the Australians as 'nature's Guinea Pigs', a sentiment accepted by anyone with whom one discusses guinea piggery. Blackie, educated to Australians by his chastening endurance test at Plymouth, and Archie the New Zealander, appreciated that every Australian who was unfortunate enough to qualify for membership of the club would be an asset; that Australian Pigs, compounded of their contrasting national characteristics of aggressive self-reliance and an underlying complex of inferiority, would relish the rankless society of the Sty. Unabashedly, Blackie and the Boss used the Australians to help them in their work and while the Australian Pigs may never have realised it, they aided greatly the general morale. Their continuing interest in the club from so far away remains an inspiration to Tom Gleave and the committee.

Among the Australian members is an Air Vice-Marshal who is recalled with particular affection by the British Pigs. Known as 'King' throughout the hospital, Adrian Cole received his injuries as Air Forward Commander in the Dieppe raid of 1942. His jaw was fractured and he collected a piece of German shell in his back when a shore battery shell landed on the bridge of the control ship, *Calpe*. From Haslar naval hospital 'King' Cole was rushed to East Grinstead, where, 'Archie had me patched up within minutes and next day, after a little forcing, agreed to have me fit in eighteen days ready to take on a Group in Northern Ireland'. Cole had impressed the need for hurry upon McIndoe because, if he could take up the appointment, he would become the first Australian to command such a large R.A.F. unit.

'King' Cole adds, 'He did this but it was so close to time that on the morning of the eighteenth day he drove me to his Harley

Street rooms, took off the bandages and dried up a large scar with methylated spirits'.

When the Australian arrived at the Sty he had asked McIndoe, 'How long will it take?' The surgeon replied, 'With bone rot and the usual troubles of fractured jaws, perhaps three to four months'. Cole replied, 'Rot, make it three weeks!'

On the eighteenth day, McIndoe whisked the Air Vice-Marshal from Harley Street to his Medical Board – which generally took two days. Cole writes, 'We got there at 10 a.m. and by 11.30 a.m. were having tea in the doctors' rest room and I took off "fit" from Northolt for Northern Ireland at 2.30 p.m. . . . Archie and I became close friends and corresponded regularly till his death. . . . I formed the opinion that Archie McIndoe was nearer to God than anyone I'd ever met in two wars and the good he did at that hospital was easily assessed by the love of his patients and the idolisation ever since.'

Through the foregoing, one may have created unintentionally, the erroneous impression that the Guinea Pig Club developed its rankless society from the easier attitude which was to be found at that time between officers and men in the Empire forces than in the British, and because McIndoe was born in New Zealand.

While a senior officer like 'King' Cole played his part in his refusal to be stuffy and the rank and file Canadians and Australians vastly helped, there was a very basic bit of British enamelware behind the growth of rankless, classless guinea piggery. A bath!

In the beginning there had been but one ward and one saline bath for burned people and into the ward and the bath came officers, men and civilians. The Salt Bath sounds magnificent, all marbled and tiled like a bath at a spa! In fact it was a very ordinary English bath, as chipped and naked as those baths one would see after an air-raid, perched among the ruins of bombed-out homes. The salt bath-room was a corner of Ward III and in there, behind ship's canvas screens on runners, a Guinea Pig could find his first relief whether he was Air Marshal or A.C.2. Tom Gleave remembers, 'They were all fried bodies to Sergeant Salmon and his orderlies who gently lowered them into the salt bath and as gently lifted them out'. Here, then, was where the rankless, classless society was born and, incidentally, where at least one Guinea Pig romance blossomed. Betty Andrews, whose duty was to help bathe pigs in the salt bath, married 'Hoke' Mahn, a legless American airman who was to die peacefully when his repair had been completed.

All ranks, all races shared in this equality and such was the spirit of wartime that the British and Empire Pigs (the Empire had not yet been processed into Commonwealth), welcomed the more warmly to club membership the Americans, one Russian and other foreign airmen who, unlucky enough to have been burned, were fortunate thereafter in their delivery to East Grinstead.

Rasumov or 'Raz' as the Pigs knew the one Russian Air Force member of the club, had been found in Germany by the Army and subsequently, delivered to East Grinstead because he had been burned and the Germans had started his plastic surgery. The question of what Raz should wear presented a unique problem. He arrived in a reach-me-down khaki battle dress and the Maestro was unwilling to approach the Russian Embassy for an appropriate Russian uniform, for fear that his patient would be collected before his surgery had been completed.

From interrogation, it appeared that Raz was the equivalent of a Flight-Lieutenant in the Red Air Force and the Pigs decided that Raz should wear the uniform and badges of a Flight-Lieutenant. Thus attired, the Russian fighter pilot accompanied his fellow Guinea Pigs to pubs, cinemas and people's homes and to many parties.

\* \* \*

'Here's your problem. Deal with it!' Not exactly the best bedside approach to the party of aircraft industrialists who were visiting the hospital and meeting Guinea Pigs for the first time. *Their* problem, as they knew it, was supplying the air force, through the Ministry of Aircraft Production, with new aircraft for the operational squadrons where men who had become Guinea Pigs, were being replaced by fresh, unscathed aircrew from the Empire air training schools. Briskly, twangily, McIndoe had thrown *his* problem at the visitors. They responded. They equipped a miniature 'factory' within the hospital, possibly the most unusual of the many little workshops which were set up in wartime Britain. A workshop where men who were trying to get what remained of their hands, to feel, to move, to clasp, to grasp again, manufactured components for the bombers and fighters which their successors and indeed some of their own number, would fly against the Germans and the Japanese.

The 'factory' was an advanced conception of occupational therapy but like the conception of the Guinea Pig Club itself, it was not the outcome of a spontaneous brain wave such as McIndoe's impressive, 'Here's your problem. Deal with it!', might suggest. It was born of two earlier mistakes and it grew into a great success because, like the club, it was an idea which fired the Pigs.

First, occupational therapy had comprised a pathetic little muster of fighter pilots knitting and rug making. Then, between surgical operations, had come the experiment of dispersing individual airmen among the aircraft factories. The former practice had proved frustrating, if not humiliating, to men who were not only smarting that they were out of the fight but also, encouraged by this type of work, beginning to see themselves as institutionalised wrecks, condemned to scarves, hearth mats and tea cosies for the rest of their lives. 'But for pleasing the Old Man, I wouldn't have done it', Geoff Page commented to Blackie.

The later workalong-side-the-workers scheme, had seemed ideal in theory but proved perilous in practice. Management took one look at the battered men, felt sorry and guilty and decided that neither money nor effort be spared to show them a good time. A Guinea Pig had to be particularly strong-minded to resist the primrose life which presented itself within and without the factory gates. Some gladly returned to their hospital beds for more reasons than that the 'slab' beckoned them to a further stage in their repair!

Blackie has criticised this scheme caustically, but it would not be fair to pass forward to his assessment of its value for Guinea Pigs in general without offering at least two slivers of evidence in support of the fact that those Pigs who bent themselves to its purpose, benefited greatly. Gordon Fredericks, the Canadian Observer who, as it will be remembered, had been burned in a Hampden crash and returned in a Mosquito to earn a bar to his Guinea Pig badge, wrote to McIndoe on June 11th, 1943, from Reid and Sigrist's electrical and aeronautical engineering factory at New Malden,

'You have seen the improvement in my hands so there is no need for me to stress the real benefit that this job has been to me on the medical side. Something that may not have been so apparent is the morale building effect of working among people who are really putting their backs into the war effort and turning out a first class product.'

And Pilot-Officer George Phillipi, the first war Colonel who had brought Smith-Barry to the Sty, received the following note at Air Ministry from Flying-Officer Mills in early 1942,

'If possible I shall be grateful if you could obtain some factory or other work for me before I return to Squadron as I shall be quite useless there really.'

Blackie's opinion of this scheme appeared in the Guinea Pig magazine,

'The Guinea Pig was packed off to a factory, generally near his home. There, unfortunately, unless he was a particularly strong-minded type and well and truly married, habits were formed which were bad. Gradually the Pig's lower nature triumphed and the situation arose of him requiring sick leave before his return from rehabilitation. Equally, M.A.P.* (aircraft factories) was not satisfactory from the factory manager's point of view. He was worried by the thought of what to do with the Guinea Pig and generally hit on the not very bright idea of treating him to life with a capital "L". The result . . . M.A.P. was not an unqualified success.'

The high life at the factories worked well enough in helping Pigs to overcome inhibitions but it was not the best way to prepare Pigs to return to service life or for resettlement. 'They lost', Blackie wrote, 'their sense of responsibility and their desire for the ordinary routine of life.'

Bringing the workshop to the hospital helped to answer this very human question because it was an action which appealed to that same spirit of guinea piggery which inspired the beginning of the club. It was an adventurous and an exclusive enterprise. Like the club and all actions which rest upon personal enthusiasm, the hospital 'factory' quickly grew into a success. Such a success that a development of the idea was to take place at a Hampshire mansion, Marchwood Park where, however, celebrating their liberation from the least disciplined hospital in Britain, some of the Pigs were to prove themselves more playful than industrious.

Jack Allaway says that after Marchwood Park, Butlins was like a home from home but upon reflection, Jack agrees with most Guinea Pigs that there are aspects of this opinion which are almost scandalously unfair to Billy Butlin! For at no Butlins would one be almost certain to find panties flying from the flag-pole and a round-the-clock performance which, as a male counter-part, would rival the high jinks of St Trinians.

*The Ministry of Aircraft Production

Marchwood Park was more than a holiday camp. It was, an Australian Pig George Taylor remembers, 'like Christmas all the time!'

The Guinea Pigs turned Marchwood into one long party, carrying to it the tradition of one aspect of the training of the Sty; an ability to withstand many wartime days and nights of partying, like the occasion when a week-long party was organised for them at the Dorchester by one of their greatest friends, Paddy Naismith.

Marchwood Park, the large Hampshire country house, takes its place in Guinea Pig history as a monument to the wild men of the Club and all the more so because the establishment of a convalescent Sty at Marchwood had been mainly brought about by the need to provide a place where the men could be gradually re-introduced to service discipline!

*     *     *

In plastic surgery cases which necessitate a long series of operations, it is very important to stay the knife between operations while the grafts settle down. The aircraft factory scheme was not to prove very satisfactory, only certain Pigs were fit enough to return, as some did, to squadron service and the hospital workshop when it started, was only available for Pigs at the hospital. McIndoe had, therefore, as he described it, become 'agitated and distracted' about this aspect of the long term treatment of severe burns.

The airmen could, possibly, have been despatched to existing service convalescent homes but the Boss did not wish to disperse them, nor to unleash them on unsuspecting staffs. He wanted them in one place where he could maintain contact and keep a fatherly eye.

Years later he revealed how Marchwood Park was achieved and in a manner wholly in keeping with the spirit of the Guinea Pig Club. He said, 'George Phillipi and I nearly ruined ourselves entertaining half the R.A.F. High Command to dinner at Claridges in order to ram Marchwood Park down their necks and especially to keep it under the control of P.5.'

However, Marchwood had an important link with East Grinstead methods. It had Johnnie Higdon, a Sergeant who became Marchwood's own Blackie and indeed, had been chosen by Blackie for the job. It may appear extraordinarily irregular that the physical training instructor who originally thought he was expected to do 'knees bend' with legless men could take his pick from the non-commissioned officers of the R.A.F. but that was the way the Guinea Pig Club operated. Short-circuiting official machinery can result in speedy arrival at the correct action and it is something at which the British, with their hawser-thick old boy network, are particularly apt. Such short cuts work best when they are supported by a powerful chief who is ready to use his friends at court to push them through. Very often the friends at court are not required. The fact that they are believed to be in the background is sufficient to pull off coups. The Guinea Pigs were not only blessed with a powerful chief in the Maestro but also with the club spirit which they themselves had generated. The combination of the two became an irresistible force and sometimes the despair of tidy-minded officials who tried to square off the paper work after the whirlwind.

Thus Blackie, when the need arose to try to introduce some semblance of the better qualities of the East Grinstead tradition at Marchwood with 'another Blackie', remembered the big, bluff Johnny Higdon whom he had met when they were sharing the incendiary task of handling the Australian airmen at Plymouth earlier in the war. With 'another Blackie', Marchwood should be kept on its toes. Or so it was hoped!

# CHAPTER NINE

'We do well to remember that the privilege of dying for one's country is not equal to the privilege of living for it.'

'Simple research has shown' Blackie wrote to a friend 'that severe burning has no effect on reproduction and the Guinea Pigs are satisfactorily holding their own biologically, if not actually increasing their numbers . . . there are many married Guinea Pigs and they have just over two children each.'

Eileen and Dickie Richardson have *exactly* two children. Twins. And if any of those unthinking people whose minds questioned Jean and Reg Hyde's fairness in breeding Piglets were to meet Heather and Keith Richardson, both seven-and-three quarters, when this story was first written, their doubts would be unconditionally dispelled.

The flames which consumed Dickie's Lancaster, after it had bombed a German panzer depot during the allied advance through Europe, not only burned away most of his face but also blinded him in both eyes. This, of course, has not prevented him contributing to the life, eyesight and handsome features of Heather and Keith – although, as Dickie says, 'You'd be surprised at the number of people who think that just because you are disfigured and blind you must be a congenital idiot'.

Nothing infuriates Dickie more than the quiet whispering between people who, because he is blind, think he cannot hear them. 'You go into a pub,' he says, 'and you hear them saying "Does he drink? Would he rather sit down?" Such people are very annoying. But I feel sorry for the other sort, the people who feel too embarrassed to talk to you. Go on a long train journey and they never say a word. I was three and a half hours on a train. One man said "Do you mind if I open the window?" and when he had left the carriage another man said "Do you mind if I shut the window?" A blind man welcomes conversation.

'Mind you now that the new plastic eyes have come in and can be fixed in the socket so that you can move them about just like real eyes it's getting easier. The new eyes are so good that sometimes people don't realise you are blind. I was on a train when another passenger offered me a paper to read. When that happens one cannot embarrass people by telling them you're blind. One simply says "No thank you very much. I've seen it".'

Dickie wonders, sometimes, how his life would have developed had the German anti-aircraft gunners not shot the 'Lanc' down. He had a very strong sense of his fortune in surviving because he was the sole survivor of the crew. He has never discovered how he escaped and, his clothes burning, floated by parachute into a French farm. Dickie was the wireless operator and he remembers hearing his pilot giving the order 'Abandon'. He was not wearing his parachute. Somehow he put it on as the bomber was blazing and stumbled towards the rear door to make his escape. But he fell flat into the flames and that is all he remembers, until he found himself on the ground and burning. His right hand, which had been almost burned away, was in a clenched position and clutching the rip cord. Dickie has no idea how he escaped from that bomber. He thinks, however, as he fell into the flames he may have been clutching at the rip cord, that perhaps there was an explosion in which he was thrown clear and in which his hand jerked his parachute open. Alternatively, another member of the crew may have picked him up and thrown him out and then failed to escape himself.

Whatever the explanation it was some time before the relatives of each member of the crew knew to which family the one survivor belonged. Identification of such a gravely burned man as Dickie was rendered the more puzzling because Dickie had taken a shower before the raid and forgotten to replace his identity disc.

Dickie was to encounter a special problem not common to the majority of sightless men. Having lost his right hand and much of the left he was without the fingers to learn braille.

However, when he returned to Worcester the Guinea Pig Club helped to establish him in a sweets and tobacco shop and he enjoyed one advantage over most people. After his pre-war employment, first as a telegraph boy and later as a postman, he would have known his way around Worcester blindfold. Unable to make use of braille or the machines which have been developed to help sightless people make notes and play them back, he began to develop a retentive memory. When a customer asked for humbugs he could go straight to the humbug jar, and he knew exactly where to find any particular brand of cigarettes. It may seem incredible, but faced with a man who was so courageously attempting to provide for himself and his family, some customers failed to play fair and Dickie's takings began to show figures which were disparate with his sales.

Thereafter, St Dunstan's trained Dickie to operate a telephone switchboard and this he has since managed with the quick darting movements which one incomplete hand demands. He has been employed as the switchboard operator at St Dunstan's near Brighton. Do not conclude that St Dunstan's gave him the job out of kindness. Dickie Richardson has been a functionally competitive switchboard operator and has been paid the rate for the job. In two respects one ventures to suggest he has been more efficient than a sighted and unmaimed operator. The memory which blindness forced upon him was to retain telephone numbers like an electronic brain and his sole aid, a tape-recorder to enable him to keep precise messages.

Although, as with J.D. and his ambition to become a forester, or Dickie's shop enterprise, it was very often believed privately that the backing of a Guinea Pig fancy might end in having to accept a losing gamble, McIndoe normally insisted upon an expert investigation before parting with a large sum of club capital or placing a strong case before the R.A.F. Benevolent Fund.

Here the club was fortunate in Alfred Wagg's acceptance of the honorary treasureship and remains indebted to the late merchant and investment banker's worldly wisdom, financial shrewdness and sense of humour; attributes which would seem to be infectious in the firm of Helbert-Wagg, since Schroeder-Wagg. Mr Harvey, who upon Alfred Wagg's retirement, succeeded him as treasurer of the club, certainly enjoyed the same attributes.

That Alfred Wagg should be living on the doorstep of the hospital was another of the unexpected advantages the club gained from the chance, as Pig legend has it, that the hospital happened conveniently to be near the school of a certain surgeon's son. Mr Wagg has not only given his financial advice to the club but also the benefit of his personal philanthropic experience, returning to the Edwardian era, when he founded the Eton Manor Club at Hackney Wick. Thus, with his usual flair for finding the best man for a job, McIndoe approached Wagg in 1943 when his thoughts were turning towards the problems of resettlement. From that time Alfred Wagg, Harvey and the merchant banking company advised the club in many individual cases.

Alfred Wagg as a banker could not, and would not, condone schemes which seemed madcap when considered away from the euphoric world of guinea piggery and in Threadneedle Street. But the treasurer having made his point never failed to follow the wishes of the club. He adhered to the club's great principle that a member should be given the chance to prove to himself what he could or could not do.

When he issued a warning, it was inevitably wrapped up in a sense of humour which is reflected in the title of his company's house journal, 'Wagtail'.

Many years ago the club consulted him upon the advisability of placing Guinea Pigs as publicans. At the end of a long and careful consideration of this question, Alfred Wagg concluded, 'I have checked with Mr Lambert, formerly my butler, whose opinion, owing to his considerable shrewdness, I have always been in the habit of asking. His comment was, "If I had all the money in the world I would not start anybody up in a pub today".'

Ignoring the warning of Alfred Wagg's butler, the Guinea Pig Club assisted several members in their endeavours to exchange their customary places 'at the bar' for the more onerous position on the other side. But Alfred's butler knew what he was about because in at least one case, that of 'Chiefy' Adams, the club experienced a certain measure of trial and tribulation before the Pig settled down as an excellent landlord at 'The Royal Oak,' Croydon, a pub which suited 'Chiefy's' personality.

* * *

Nobody at the annual dinner could remember very much about Roy Lane. Joe Biel, the Pole sitting opposite, said he had never heard of him. Blind Dickie Richardson, waiting for Joe to finish cutting up a portion of turkey, could not recall a Pig of that name. But John Banham, large and executive-looking, a Battle of Britain fighter pilot who became a brewer, thought back to 1940 and 1941. 'Very early. Yes, we called him Lulu. Apart from that I cannot tell you much. Nice chap. Does Tom know?' Tom Gleave did not know.

Squadron-Leader Lane was a forgotten Guinea Pig, but he merits more than passing acknowledgement as a member of the club, partly because he was one of the intrepid Pigs who, after repair at the Sty, returned to operations and subsequently lost their lives; partly because the manner of 'Lulu' Lane's arrival at East Grinstead, though unremembered by his fellow Pigs, is among the more memorable of Guinea Pig exploits. And partly because, after almost losing a leg on the operation table, and despite his wounds and burns, he walked through the jungles of Burma alongside Bernard Fergusson of the Chindits.

But Roy Lane's story begins on August 26th, 1940, when his Hurricane squadron was ordered to intercept a raid approaching Portsmouth. Roy's story of what happened that day is, as a contemporary description by a Battle of Britain pilot worthy of the telling. As a qualification for membership of the Guinea Pig Club it is unique.

'We climbed to the height ordered on the course and presently we sighted two formations of thirty Heinkels, each protected by roughly fifty ME 109s. We carried out the normal head-on attack, but in this instance the bombers didn't break their formation, and it was our squadron that had to break instead, thereby scattering our aircraft all over the sky.

'I continued my attack too long and had to break off underneath the bombers, coming out the other end among their fighters. I managed to get straight through this lot without any of them attacking me and I climbed straight up again to get in a better position to attack the bombers. As I did so I noticed that one bomber formation was leaving and heading back towards the coast of France. These bombers were still a considerable height above me which meant that I had to climb as fast as I could. . . . Behind the bombers were about five or six ME 110 fighters, and as I was directly below them I thought they would probably not see me as I attacked the bombers. I took a good chance on this, keeping a sharp look-out in my mirror. Unfortunately as I was about to open fire on a bomber – and due to the fact that I was unable to take any evasive action – one of the Nazi fighters got me in his sights and my plane was hit in the engine. I heard two loud explosions and I guessed I'd been hit pretty badly. As I pushed the cockpit cover back I passed out through lack of oxygen. My oxygen apparatus had been badly damaged when my plane was hit.

'As I fainted I saw a dim red glow in front of my eyes – but I didn't understand what this was until I came to at a lower altitude.

'I found that my Hurricane was not only on fire but was diving upside down. Luckily I was hanging by my straps, which enabled me to keep my face out of the flames a good deal. Even so I was unable to open my eyes due to the intense heat and I tried to operate the quick release pin so that I could fall out of the aircraft and use my parachute. For some reason this didn't work so I tried rolling my plane right way up. But this was unsuccessful, due to the rolling motion of the aircraft blowing the flames still hotter. Eventually I got so tired of struggling to get out, and I was so frightened, that I just "gave up the ghost" and I really began to think I was in hell.

'Shortly after this – I don't know how long after – I realised that things were much cooler. So I opened my eyes – to find there was no aeroplane around me. I think that the straps must have burned through, allowing me to fall out. I didn't wait long to admire the scenery, but began to see about opening my parachute. On looking around I discovered that it wasn't on me. As I knew I had it when I started I began to think it had been burned off me, but through force of habit I put my right arm on my left hip where the rip-cord should be and I found something there. I gave it the hell of a tug, and then there was a violent crack and the canopy opened. I quickly discovered that I was upside down in the parachute, suspended by the ankles. Either the shoulder straps had burned through, or they came off when I was struggling to get out of the plane. At all events I was falling upside down with the harness of the chute entangled in my flying boots. I was very glad indeed that I had on a pair of boots that fitted me well.

'For some reason I wanted to take my gloves and helmet off. The helmet and left hand glove came off all right, but my right hand glove was burned and shrivelled on to my hand which had been in the flames most of the time. I managed finally to get that glove off, but unfortunately a lot of skin came off with it, leaving my hand very raw indeed. Then I tried to right myself into the harness, but to no avail. I just couldn't do it.

'I noticed I was drifting over a small town, but I don't remember a great lot about the descent, as I was in a very shocked condition, to say nothing of being badly frightened. I did notice, however, that I seemed to be heading for a ploughed field, and despite the fact that I was due to land upside down with a shock comparable to a jump from a height of nineteen feet I thought I might get away with it.

'As I came lower I could see in the corner of the field a man and his wife (at least I expected it was his wife) and I felt glad that I should be able to get such immediate help. I prepared for the

107

landing, and protected myself as best I could in my upside-down position by winding my arms around my head and by arching my body away from the direction of travel so that I could land on my left shoulder.

'I hit the ground and opened my eyes to see that I was at least alive and that I was being dragged along the ground by the parachute. I managed to collapse it, then I sat up to release myself from the harness. When I had managed this I stood up, fully expecting the man and woman to come to help me, but they didn't. They just stood still near the house, looking at me, and probably thinking that it was just another example of R.A.F. high spirits.

'I started to march over to them with the intention of telling them just what I thought of their behaviour, but I hadn't got very far before there was a lot of violent shouting. I looked round and saw about twenty Army types barging through the hedge with fixed bayonets, very excited soldiery telling me to so-and-so stop where I was. This annoyed me even more. I just stood and swore at them from A to Z, which convinced them that I was friendly and British. A Corporal came up and asked me rather stupidly if I was hurt, which question seemed to me – in view of the fact that I was limping badly, my hand was cooked, my face was red with burns, any my right trouser leg was burned off – superfluous to say the least.

'However, with the Corporal's help, I managed to limp down to the road by the edge of the field, where one of the men had stopped a private car. In this car were two old ladies, one of which climbed out and asked me politely whether I would prefer to sit in the front or the back. I regret to say that I told her that I didn't so-and-so mind where I so-and-so well sat.

'That was about all there was to it. I was driven to an Army casualty station where I was given first aid, then I was sent to the squadron's favourite hospital where I met three of the other fellows who had been shot down in the same fight.'

After repair Roy Lane experienced a quiet spell, quiet that was by comparison with his descent head-first and with what was to follow in Burma. He toured the aircraft factories giving pep talks to workers. Production figures improved in the wake of a badly burned but articulate airman and such visits brought a reciprocal benefit to a Guinea Pig in the sense of a continuing contribution to the war effort; and even more important to a badly injured man, a feeling of being needed and a consequent restoration of confidence.

Touring the factory benches and speaking to the assembled workers in their canteens began to pall, however, when a Pig's physical strength had returned. Like so many of the Pigs who, well repaired, considered they should make an early return to operational flying, Roy Lane grew impatient for a cockpit. The unit he now joined was no ordinary squadron. It was the Merchant Ship Fighter Unit at Speke near Liverpool – the unit which supplied Hurricane fighters and pilots for the catapult apparatus which was beginning to appear on the decks of the merchant ships carrying war supplies between the United States, Britain and Russia. Granted but a fractional chance of survival once they had been catapulted from a ship which was beyond Hurricane range of land, the Catafighters accompanied the Atlantic and Russian convoys to counteract the preying four-engined Focke-Wulf Condor reconnaissance-bombers which were directing the U-Boat packs towards the allied convoys. Roy Lane survived several voyages, before returning ashore to command a small fighter station established near Archangel, to provide fighter cover for the convoys as they approached Russia.

However, considering the serious injuries and burns he had received in the Battle of Britain and that at one moment the amputation of his right leg had rested on McIndoe's decision, it is the next and final phase in this forgotten Guinea Pig's career which is the most remarkable.

Posted to India, he volunteered to march into Burma and operate behind the Japanese lines with the Chindits, serving as an air liaison officer to Brigadier Bernard Fergusson. When Fergusson and his Chindits reached their area of operations they built an air strip in the heart of Japanese-held country, and a Hurricane was flown in for Lane's use. Later, he had flown to India to liaise on air support and was returning to the jungle air strip when his Hurricane developed engine trouble. He forced-landed some twenty miles east of the Chindwin river and the R.A.F. dropped his food, maps and news of enemy depositions in the area. The Japanese found him and, it is believed, beheaded him. Bernard Fergusson wrote from India. 'It seemed hard that he should be missing as a result of engine failure after all his escapes in the Battle of Britain and over the Arctic convoys.'

\* \* \*

The scene at the annual dinner of the Guinea Pig Club, as it appears to the uninitiated, has been set previously: Centre piece of the annual 'Lost Weekend' which, with the passing of the years is losing its 'lostness' it nevertheless manages to produce new legends for the Guinea Pig repertoire and to add lustre to some of the old ones.

Thus, when Freeman Strickland, one of the Australian Pigs, attended a dinner in 1956, the Maestro recalled, 'You will remember that Strick has quite a reputation as a souvenir hunter. When he was here during the war, he managed to "find" quite a lot of things that took his fancy – why, he even managed to remove a stag's head from the walls of this very hotel. . . .

'Whenever I couldn't find anything in my house, I was pretty sure that Strick had taken a fancy to it, and that the missing article was floating around Australia somewhere.

'It was whispered that Strick had to pay excess freight on something like half-a-ton of stuff . . .'

Replying Strick said, 'I was somewhat disgusted when I got home to find that the market value of the souvenirs was way below anything I had hoped.'

After breakfast next morning, the Maestro encountered the vast Lobster sign which adorns 'Ye Olde Felbridge Hotel' inside his front door.

Strickland and his fellow Australian, Ken Gilkes, had succeeded in combining a demonstration that they had not lost their touch with an inimitably Australian expression of their gratitude to their host for the traditional party, which began at his home after the Dinner had broken up and continued into the early hours of the following morning. Connie McIndoe lives no longer in her beautiful Millwood Manor near East Grinstead, but she maintains the tradition, pitching a giant marquee near the hospital. 'Connie's Big Top' as she calls it!

Reuniting annually, the Guinea Pigs – so many of whom were little more than schoolboys when an ambulance brought them to the Sty – discard the creased attitudes which family life, divorce, rent, rates and sometimes alimony, have laden them and rediscover the prangy humour which nourished them mentally when they had been 'fried'. Some have been known to book for the dinner but never to reach it, the first day of the reunion having proved *too* convivial. Then, they are put to bed in a ward and are as much, if not more at home, as those who have survived until the dinner.

Among those who stayed the course of the 1952 dinner was the Guinea Pig Air Marshal, Dick Atcherley. Thanking Archie, he wrote of the club, 'It's a wonderful movement and I never cease to be inspired and uplifted when I depart – this time to such effect that I knocked down a wall. But it is the most eloquent tribute to your personal leadership and work.'

However, with the years the annual weekend has grown more sedate. Never again will so few Guinea Pigs aggregate such vast consumption as at the 1949 dinner when a count established the astonishing fact that 225 Guinea Pigs had consumed 3,000 bottles of beer and 125 bottles of whisky, in addition to six dozen bottles of sherry presented by the Spanish Embassy.

Although the reputation of the original Ward III 'grogging club' is by no means let down, the 'Lost Weekend' is beginning to take on a family aspect, the very prospect of which would have horrified some of the same Pigs fifteen years ago. Wives and children and now grandchildren abound and the medical and welfare check-up presided over by Blackie and Russell is taken most seriously. If not always on behalf of the Pigs, then on behalf of their families. But the spirit in which even welfare matters are approached is hearty and convivial. Thus, one finds during the Boss's lifetime, a surgeon writing about Reg Hyde's son Peter, then two.

'Dear Sir Archibald McIndoe, This little boy's mother tells me that at a Guinea Pig dinner you told his father that you would arrange his further treatment.'

Back went the characteristic reply, 'This patient's father is a Guinea Pig and well known to me. At the last reunion he told me a story about his child which was not nearly so clear as your very full note . . . I cannot at this moment remember what I said as the occasion was a fairly convivial one, but I have now written to the boy's father telling him that he should certainly continue under your care.'

And there was the cosmetic operation which the Maestro was never to perform on Patsy, Sandeman-Allen's little girl, whose father wrote to Russell, 'Last year Archie promised to see Patsy this year and do a "cosmetic" job on her ears which stick out through her hair'. At E.G. the promise was kept.

The annual dinner of the Guinea Pig Club, though growing yearly more sedate, is always 'convivial', to re-employ the Boss's description of the 1957 occasion. In his lifetime the President of the club, more of a Chief Executive than a President, worked minutely to make the 'Lost Weekend' both smooth and convivial.

One finds him writing to Blackie in 1951, 'I think the badge is pretty roughly made (former Guinea Pig badge), but what can you expect for 1/7d? . . . Now as to the dinner menu which will be simple, homely, but good – Steak, Kidney and Oyster pudding with brussels sprouts and cream potatoes. This is to be carefully compounded, tasted and scrutinised by John Hunter himself. . . . I have no further views about the guest of honour. This is very difficult. If we ask any of the big new wigs, nobody will know them, and they won't know anybody. On the other hand there's no accounting for the way retired R.A.F. officers seem to sink into senility the moment they are out of uniform . . .'.

The annual dinner, formerly set in the Whitehall at East Grinstead, in the bar of which presided over by the Guinea Pigs' great friend Bill Gardiner, so many Pigs had re-discovered that they could laugh and drink, although it sometimes necessitated drinking beer through a rubber tube, has removed to the more pretentious Ye Olde Felbridge Hotel. The beloved Whitehall, second shrine of guinea piggery after Ward III, fell under the property hammer and sadly is no more. Flowers, the brewers, built a new pub near the hospital and named it The Guinea Pig, but, gesture though this was, the bricky pub is no compensation for the old Whitehall with all its memories. The erasure of the Whitehall, the roadhouse decor of Ye Olde Felbridge, the use of The Guinea Pig as a grogging HQ only on Lost Weekends – all serve to remind one of what, apart from the 'Lost' attributes of the weekend, and the welfare and medical soundings, pulls several hundred of the war's most badly injured men to East Grinstead every autumn.

It is a pilgrimage for a renewal of faith to a place which, through its refusal from the very beginning in 1940 to show that it thought there was anything different about Guinea Pigs, contributed as much to their recovery as Blackie, Russell, John Hunter or the Boss himself. East Grinstead.

# CHAPTER TEN

'Our Club . . . more exclusive than Boodles, Bucks, Whites and the Royal Yacht Squadron rolled into one.'

Derek Crane was in a motor torpedo boat when it blew up at sea. One of the first impressions after the naval sick-berth attendants had delivered him from Harwich was that few inland places could be less nautical than East Grinstead. It was not simply that a sailor was a rarity among the light blue 'jobs' at the hospital. Something else was missing. Naval discipline.

The boisterous irreverence which buoyed up the Guinea Pigs, the fearlessness of authority, the friendliness regardless of rank or rating, the calculated carelessness of normal service good order and discipline – it all disquieted Derek Crane. It was a situation as removed from his experience as was East Grinstead in population, clangour and seaport odour from Devonport, Portsmouth or Chatham. After several months in this very different environment, the sailor's first feelings of disquiet had improved to nothing better than bewilderment.

So many years later his chief early memory of his arrival at the hospital is his astonishment when a sergeant told the surgeon who was about to examine him, 'Jerry, we've got a new patient.' Jerry was Squadron-Leader Jerry Moore, a very great favourite with the Pigs, especially those whose hands came under his 'chop' on the 'slab'. Hands were Jerry Moore's speciality.

Derek Crane never really understood his Air Force companions, but the airmen decided that this badly burned sailor, being an odd-man-out in the company of the odd needed a strong tot of guinea piggery. As a seaman he qualified even less than little George Hindley for membership of the Club. But like Johnny Hill and Little George he was accepted as another 'exception to the aircrew rule'.

Undoubtedly there will be non-aircrew former Service patients of the Queen Victoria Hospital who will read this and complain that they were not invited to join the Guinea Pig Club with Crane and his fellow 'exceptions to the rule'. There was, for example, one airman whose injuries brought him to East Grinstead and who was at first indignant when his application was turned down. Subsequently he accepted refusal of membership gracefully. 'I was not aircrew . . . I was not a burns case' he wrote to Russell Davies. 'Further . . . my injuries were small with me only falling off a pushbike.' Those not created Life Pigs as 'exceptions' must accept that the Guinea Pig Club gathered to its bosom non-aircrew airmen and others whose personal fortitude, need and company at the Sty have inspired their admission.

But the Guinea Pig Club could never have attained its unique position as a club 'more exclusive than Boodles, Bucks, Whites and the Royal Yacht Squadron rolled into one' without the generously impulsive nature with which Maxillonians and others from the fighter squadrons endowed it and which McIndoe fostered. Indeed he could not fail but to foster it because, in so doing, he was creating the Club in the image of an aspect of his own character; an aspect of which he was sharply reminded by the member who, mixed up in a Guinea Pig controversy, wrote to him, 'My dear old Archie, We all have our failings . . . so pardon me if I tell you that one of yours is your habit of rushing your hurdles, of leaping before you look, of going off half-cocked. It is a good fault that we all accept because it does so much more good than the general negative bluntness of most of the people of today. It's part of you as a very successful, dynamic character whom we all so greatly admire.'

Like converts to a faith or a political party, the 'exceptions' strengthened their club. Derek Crane, George Hindley, and the other exceptions, contributed substantially towards this rare survival of the nineteen forties – the continuity of a wartime cameraderie and purpose.

Generally, when Service people go their separate ways to the top, to the middle, to the bottom of civilian life, the former cameraderie, the shared anxieties, are submerged by new loyalties, new fears. Sooner or later the best intentioned promises unfailingly to reunite founder among new responsibilities at home and at work. Like old soldiers, reunions fade away. But the 'exceptions to the rule' are the keenest reuniters, partly because like George Hindley they are so very conscious and grateful of what the club has done for them. Their gratitude and enthusiasm helps to cement the brickwork of Tom Gleave, Blackie, Russell, Bernard Arch, his colleague Phil Barrowman, and Henry Standen and Sam Gallop, present and past editors of the Guinea Pig Magazine.

The existence of the 'exceptions' serves to emphasise another aid to the unusual factor of the club's survival so many years after blood and fire and frost had brought its members together. This was that although the majority of members were aircrew, and 'fried', they had little in common.

Most clubs, because they *are* clubs, contain members who share a common interest, common knowledge, common pleasures or who are by profession, background or environment, pleased enough with one another to hoist the unkindly blackball against those whom they rate outside their personal orbit. But the Pigs were unglamorous 'erks', shop assistants like J.D. and Tommy Brandon, insurance clerks like Les Syrett, bank clerks like Pip Parratt, high ranking regular officers like Dick Atcherley and 'King' Cole, almost straight-from-school boys like Owen-Smith and many others. Nothing in common here.

It was Pip Parratt who emphasised this nothing-in-common aspect, possibly because he is proudly conscious of his promotion to Flight-Lieutenant from the lower reaches of life in a bank. He returned to the bank and like Derek Crane and Henry Standen, he was another very badly hurt man who lived in East Grinstead, close to the Sty. He would have liked to have remained in the Service but accepts that he is lucky enough to be alive after falling from eighteen thousand feet inside a blazing, crashing Lancaster bomber which broke its back across a line of wagons in a Hamburg railway yard. Pip maintains his connection with the Service, however, by parading regularly as a member of the Royal Observer Corps and instructing Air Training cadets – sometimes to the chagrin of his wife, who as Olwen Gregory was a nurse at the hospital. She considers that Pip has done enough for his country and could spare himself long nights out in cold observation posts.

When the Germans found Pip's body in the wreckage of the Lancaster and the railway wagons they pulled it out into the snow, rolled it over among the railway lines, and thought it was dead. Madness, the enemy said, for these heavy bombers to attempt a daylight raid. Well, here was another Englishman who had asked for trouble. He was dead and who could say that he had not deserved it.

It was fortunate for Pip that the first Germans who found him thought no man could have survived such a crash. He heard later that, of those who had managed to bale out, the Flight Engineer had been shot on the end of his parachute and the rest of the crew beaten and kicked by German civilians until some members of the Luftwaffe arrived on the scene and stopped them.

When they had repaired Flight-Lieutenant 'Pip' Parratt, D.F.M., at the Sty and equipped him with a hefty surgical boot to offset his crippling injuries, they returned him to his civilian occupation in a bank.

Pip is the most cheerful and helpful of tellers but there are times, one senses, when he wonders whether his injuries have retarded, if not killed, his chances of promotion and regrets the Royal Air Force career that might have developed had he been fit enough to seek to remain, after hostilities, as a regular.

Where one encounters regret, and very occasionally a touch of bitterness, one cannot conclude – as one had expected to conclude before receiving the privilege of their confidence – that the feelings are born of the Pig's sense of misfortune. They come, one learns, from subsequent frustration which, while related to the origin of their disability, develops when life does not seem to be going too well or if a Pig feels cheated of opportunities and business promotion.

Invariably in serious conversation – and this in some cases can only be attained after one has gained sufficient of the Pig's confidence to break through the Guinea Pig banter barrier – ('Did anyone tell you of the time Tubby Taylor . . . Only "drinking" wigs are worn at the dinner. . . . What about the time Johnny Higdon took us from Marchwood to Bournemouth and Dixie Dean brought back the keep-off-the-grass signs. . . . Or the night John Hunter drank Clark Gable under the table?') – invariably, a Pig will reflect upon his lost opportunity in the Air Force. Not, in this context, from the wartime concern for fighting the enemy, but as a career.

Obviously the Royal Air Force in peacetime could not have retained all the aircrew officers who might have wished to remain in the service or to return to it, once dissatisfied with civilian life. There are, however, Pigs who *think* they would happily exchange their seats in the bus to the office with Jackie Hutchinson, the Guinea Pig who remained aircrew or Captain Jack Mann who flew with Middle East Airlines. Certainly, neither Hutchinson nor Mann would wish the reverse!

This recurring 'dream' can be unsettling.

Service as aircrew opened a frontier to so many of the Pigs, airmen like J.D., the draper's assistant from Scotland, Sid McQuillan the Yorkshire colliery clerk, Dickie Richardson, a whistling telegraph boy who knew Worcester inside out – on his red bicycle. As Dickie said, he never dreamed of 'joining those who-go-out-to-dinner,' and when it happened, his mother who had been in private service, told him: 'Don't worry, just start with the cutlery on the outside, and eat your way inwards. Then you can't make a mistake.' But, at first, Dickie was terrified he would.

Understandably this sense of 'I wonder-what-might-have-been' is stronger among those to whom their new found public respect and social elevation as aircrew n.c.o.s and commissioned officers came as a pleasant surprise and contrast than among those who like Richard Hillary and Tom Gleave were more accustomed to it. André Browne, for example, wartime Flying-Officer and Typhoon fighter pilot, had to endure a most humble, monotonous and poorly paid occupation until Blackie recently rescued him.

With André the club's resettlement task was not made any simpler by the Pig's belief that, being half Belgian his broken accent was against him. There was no reason why it should have been but André had got it into his head that, as he said, 'In the war a foreign accent was glamorous. Now one is just a dirty little foreigner with a bad pair of hands.' The Club's emphasis upon the demands of social disability is clearly illustrated by André's case. He resents the loss of confidence which belonged to him when he sewed on his pilot's wings. 'I am all right' he says 'until I notice that whoever I am talking to has seen my hands, and his eyes keep returning to them. Then I freeze and my foreign accent becomes all the more pronounced.'

Sid McQuillan, after the especial esprit of ferrying supplies to the *maquis*, was restless as a clerk until through his personal effort and enterprise he attained an executive position in the Kent coalfield.

Freddie Whitehorn, more seriously burned than Bertram Owen-Smith who was at the controls of the same bomber when, with the two Pig pilots aboard on a conversion training flight, engine trouble enforced a crash landing, says, 'Returning to nine to five office work after captaining a bomber seemed most unattractive'.

Freddie, then a Sergeant-Pilot, was one of the young men who in 1938 had found adventurous release from clerking as a weekend volunteer. He has kept an interest in the Air Force, through an elder son in the service, and a spare time appointment as Pilot-Officer in the Air Training Corps.

But there are members of the club who brood quietly – and occasionally burst out angrily – that their injuries have held them back in civilian life, that the Air Force unwrapped their potential and would have provided them with a career in which their abilities would have been used. That this sense exists is recognised by the club, particularly by Blackie and Russell, both of whom are always ready to do what they can to go to the root of such problems and help to re-settle a Guinea Pig if such a course is considered to be desirable. *Their* problem is that not every Pig realises how he can be advised in this very personal direction and Blackie suspects that privately a number of Pigs may be nursing an unnecessary discontent. On the other hand it is equally understandable that the clerk, say in an office, who does not wish to admit to himself that he might never in any circumstances, have made a manager, might prefer to harbour to himself the excuse of his wartime injuries for finding himself passed over.

It may seem a cruel conclusion but the saying that some men are more equal than others cannot be overlooked even when discussing such hurt men. In general, the play-safers – not of course in the sense in which they fought the enemy and were decorated for courage – would have been happier in the Service with their newly-discovered social distinction and technical talents, burned or unburned. Equally the enterprising, burned or unburned would have found achievement in or out of the Service, as have some members of the Guinea Pig Club.

Leaving aside such considerations, one truth is positive, however well, ordinarily, or badly, Guinea Pigs may have fared since they left the Sty. It is that many of them would have been sunk without the spirit of guinea piggery.

Lecturing students during the war McIndoe said, 'The suicide rate among them might be very high were it not for the fact that the right method of dealing with them is to get them out, not to treat them as people to be put behind screens.' And all done by the spirit of guinea piggery without the prop of a 'trick cyclist'. No psychiatrist was employed residentially at the Sty.

The correctness of McIndoe's creed is daily demonstrated by members of the Guinea Pig Club who are engaged in competitive life. For, while most Guinea Pigs do not care to recall such feelings, Bernard Arch, the hospital's R.A.F. clerk who became

118

the club's honorary organising secretary, writes:

'The severely disfigured patient faced an abrupt change in his very personality. From knowing what he looked like and how he faced the world, he was thrown into a situation where he was not even sure of his own appearance from day to day. He expected and sought, the look of horror, or at best compassion, in the eyes of the normal person. Frequently unable to eat, or drink, or converse normally, owing to scar formation round the mouth, certain natures became morose and tended to shun all social contact. Others became unnaturally aggressive, apparently glorying in their power to shock, but suffering profound mental agonies in the darkness of the night.'

Without their club, The Guinea Pig Club, many of the war's most seriously injured airmen would never have left institutional life and neither the play-safers nor the commercially daring would have had the opportunity to exist or to thrive in competitive civilian life; or to keep their tail-less end up in the pensions war which continues.

For, with the loss of Archie, the Boss, the Maestro, their Father, the Guinea Pigs turned more than ever to the club – 'one of the curiosities of the war'. The club became the mother of them all, their security and their someone-to-go-to.

# THE GUINEA PIGS

J. Adamczyk
J. G. Adams
R. R. Adams
R. Adcock
H. Aldridge
J. A. Allard
J. Allaway
G. W. Allen
T. Allen
K. Allison
H. Anderson
I. Anderson
J. Anderson
J. A. Anderson
L. Anderson
J. R. Andrew
W. G. Anglin
J. P. Angold
R. I. Armstrong
J. D. Ashton
D. J. Aslin
R. L. R. Atcherley
M. R. Atherton
J. C. Atkinson
D. Bacon
R. Bagard
J. H. Bain
A. R. Ball
R. J. Ball
F. A. Ballentyne
A. J. Banham
V. Banks
W. D. Barber
J. S. Barker
A. A. Barrow
P. Barry
K. M. Base
G. E. Beauchamp
W. Begbie

J. Benbow
G. C. Bennett
G. H. Bennions
G. H. Bernier
N. E. Berrington-
    Pickett
L. E. Berryman
M. Biddle
J. Biel
F. Bielawski
H. Bird-Wilson
J. B. W. Birks
M. Bobitlo
C. Boissonas
D. E. B. Bond
H. Van Dyke Bonney
W. J. Bourn
A. C. Bowes
W. M. Bowyer
C. I. L. Boyd
G. P. Bradley
P. F. Branch
T. W. Brandon
K. Branston
C. Briggs
E. Bristow
R. Broadbent
E. Bronski
P. W. S. Brooke
R. H. Brooke
N. Brooks
J. Broughton
T. Brown
A. H. R. Browne
K. Browne
T. Browne
E. Brunskill
J. D. Bubb
J. W. Buckee

F. G. Buckle
H. W. Buckman
V. G. Bull
E. G. Buller
F. Bullock
G. Burrell
W. G. Burton
G. Butcher
J. C. Butler
M. W. Buttler
L. Caddell
B. S. Cadman
E. A. Cain
L. Cameron
B. Campbell
C. Campbell
K. Cap
J. Capka
J. Carlier
E. L. Carlsen
R. Carnall
E. M. Cartwright
L. P. Catellier
E. Cecille
E. Chapman
M. Charbonneau
R. W. H. Charles
C. Chater
L. E. Chiswell
R. G. Chitham
G. B. Clarke
J. R. Clarke
R. Clarkson
R. Cleland
J. Clifford
J. Colbert
A. T. Cole
J. Cole
L. P. H. Cole

G. Collier
R. Collin
R. Colyar
J. Condon
A. Cooke
C. Cooper
K. G. Cooper
W. Cooper
M. Coote
F. Coppock
A. Corpe
L. R. Corrigan
W. Cowham
J. W. Craig
S. Crampton
D. Crane
D. Crauford
H. R. Crombie
W. G. J. Cruickshank
J. Cummins
W. Cunningham
H. Curwain
G. Dakin
R. W. Dalkin
E. D. Dash
C. E. Davidson
K. Davidson
F. S. Davies
K. Davies
J. Davis
P. Davoud
F. G. Davy
E. J. Davy
R. L. F. Day
F. J. Dean
L. Dean
K. B. L. Debenham
G. De Bruyn
H. J. Dee
E. J. De Lyon
A. Deniall
T. Derenzy
Mohamed
  Dermerdash
F. Devers
W. Dewar
W. A. Douglas

G. Dove
O. Dove
E. A. Doyle
W. Doyle
A. S. Dredge
G. Dufort
G. Duncan
J. W. Duncan
R. D. Dunscombe
P. Edmond
G. Edmonds
Wm. Edmonston
G. D. Edwards
H. Edwards
A. Elkes
P. R. Ellis
Nedim Erakdogan
H. Ernst
J. Evans
J. Everett
H. Fairclough
F. Falkiner
G. R. Fawcett
E. Ferguson
J. Ferguson
S. G. Finnemore
G. Figuiere
K. Fisher
P. H. Fitz-Gerald
J. Fleming
G. Forbes
M. E. Forster
G. L. Fowler
R. P. Fowler
W. J. Foxley
R. A. Fraser
R. Fraser
R. G. Fredericks
D. Freehorn
H. M. Friend
S. R. Gallop
R. Gambier-Parry
A. H. Gambling
T. A. Garne
R. Garvin
R. Gauvin
V. P. Gerald

F. G. Gibbs
C. Gilkes
J. Gillies
J. Gingles
G. B. Giradet
S. Given
T. P. Gleave
J. Glebocki
D. R. Glossop
N. W. Glover
W. Golding
C. E. Goodman
L. A. Goodson
J. F. Gourlay
R. Graham
A. Graveley
H. T. Green
J. Grill
J. Grudzien
J. N. Gunnis
E. Gwardiak
J. Haddock
L. Haines
N. D. Hallifax
D. Hall
K. Hall
F. Hanton
J. Harding
C. Harper
J. Harrington
W. W. Harris
L. R. W. Harrison
K. Harrop
P. R. Hart
D. Harvey
F. R. Haslam
L. E. Hastings
A. J. Hawksworth
W. Heine
D. A. Helsby
A. J. Henderson
A. C. Henry
J. Heslop
G. Hewison
R. J. Hewitt
W. R. Hibbert
C. Hicks

D. Hicks
J. Hicks
W. J. Higgins
E. Hiley
J. P. Hill
N. Hill
W. Hill
R. Hillary
A. J. Hills
G. J. Hindley
C. Hitchcock
V. R. Hobbs
W. W. Hocken
C. G. S. Hodgkinson
R. Holdsworth
R. H. Holland
N. P. C. Holmes
N. Holmes
W. Holmes
J. Hood
J. Hooper
R. Houston
F. Hubbard
J. Hughes
J. D. E. Hughes
W. S. Humphreys
D. W. Hunt
C. O. Hunter
C. A. L. Hurry
G. W. Hutchinson
W. J. Hutchinson
R. H. J. Hyde
K. Intepe
N. L. Ireland
G. E. Jackson
J. W. F. Jacob
G. T. Jarman
J. Jarman
C. R. Jenkins
G. R. Johnston
B. Jones
I. M. Jones
I. W. Jones
J. S. Jones
O. Jones
F. Keeno
J. Keep

J. H. F. Kemp
F. P. King
J. Kerr
B. Kingcome
J. Kirby
J. J. Knott
W. Knowles
W. P. Korwell
J. Koukall
E. Krasnodembski
P. S. Kyd
E. LaCasse
N. Lambell
E. G. Lancaster
D. Lanctot
A. Lander
R. Lane
W. Lane
N. C. Langham-
    Hobart
A. Landland
S. Langley
G. Lawson
G. T. Lea
R. G. F. Lee
S. M. Lee
T. M. Lee
A. Leitch
J. Lestanges
R. Leupp
E. J. Lever
J. Levi
B. Levin
W. H. Liddiard
E. S. Lightley
M. Lipsett
R. T. Lloyd
E. S. Lock
B. Loneon
S. Loosley
A. J. Lord
R. C. Lord
G. J. Lowe
J. Lowe
S. Lugg
D. M. Lunney
L. Lymburner

J. McBride
O. J. McCabe
R. C. McCallum
A. McConnell
S. MacCormac
G. McCully
T. McGovan
R. A. McGowan
B. McHolm
I. C. S. McIvor
T. D. McKeown
J. McLaughlin
C. MacLean
C. A. McLeod
D. McNally
D. C. McNeill
A. C. H. Maclean
J. F. MacPhail
W. J. MacPherson
S. McQuillan
D. McTavish
R. Major
J. Mann
J. Marceau
J. Marcotte
Cyril Marjoram
J. Marshall
D. D. Martin
J. Martin
S. Martin
W. Martin
W. Martin
D. C. Marygold
R. M. Mathieson
J. Mathis
J. W. Maxwell
J. May
L. Melling
J. C. Melvill
W. R. Methven
J. Miles
N. E. Miles
W. H. Mills
B. Mitchell
S. R. Molivadas
E. G. S. Monk
J. F. Montgomery

M. Montpetit
O. G. Moore
F. S. Moores
J. Mordue
A. Morgan
I. C. A. Morris
H. J. Morson
M. H. Mounsdon
G. D. Mufford
J. G. E. Munt
G. D. I. Neale
R. G. Nelson
A. Nesbitt
B. P. Nettleton
N. Newman
W. Newson
T. Nichols
N. Nisbet
J. Nivison
B. R. Noble
G. Noble
W. L. Noble
R. Noon-Ward
C. T. Norman
S. A. Noyes
J. B. O'Brien
D. O'Connell
K. O'Connor
H. Ogden
T. O'Halloran
E. Orchel
G. Orman
D. O'Sullivan
F. Overeijnder
E. Owen
A. G. Page
R. B. Pape
H. E. Parratt
A. Paszkowski
R. H. Payne
T. J. Peach
E. G. Pearce
G. H. Pearce
R. E. Pearce
A. Pearson
H. Peel
J. K. Kelly

F. Penman
P. Pereuse
E. J. Perry
D. Petit
H. Phillips
L. Phillips
S. A. Piercy
D. Pike
J. Pitts
M. A. Platsko
T. A. Podbereski
E. Poole
J. Poole
K. L. Porter
R. F. Pretty
D. Price
B. Propas
A. Proudlove
D. M. Pryor
F. J. Quigley
I. MacP. Quilter
G. H. Raby
R. Ralston
H. J. Randall
R. F. G. Raphael
V. Rasumov
R. Tatajczak
J. Redekopp
J. Reece
C. G. Reynolds
G. Reynolds
J. Reynolds
S. Reynolds
C. Rhodes
D. B. Richardson
W. Richardson
J. Rickard
B. Ridding
F. T. Rix
E. J. Robbins
J. L. Roberson
E. D. Roberts
R. Roberts
T. J. Roberts
A. B. Robertson
J. H. Rogers
S. Round

A. Rowley
A. Royds
J. H. Russell
K. Russell
J. St. John
J. F. M. Sampson
J. A. Sandeman-
    Allen
A. C. Saunders
R. T. Saunders
J. H. Schloesing
T. J. Scoffield
E. E. Scott
J. E. Scott
G. R. Scott-Farnie
D. R. Scrivens
R. Shallis
A. Shankland
W. Shankland
W. Simms
D. W. Simpson
J. H. Simpson
W. Simpson
J. A. Sims
A. Siska
L. Skoczylas
B. O. Smith
D. B. Smith
J. Smith
J. C. Smith
P. C. Smith
P. S. S. Smith
R. Smith-Barry
R. J. Smith
T. A. Smith
T. C. F. Smith
T. G. Smith
W. E. Smith
K. C. Smyth
A. B. Snelling
K. Snyder
L. J. Somers
J. Southwell
G. L. Spackman
W. R. Speedie
B. Spooner
W. H. C. Spooner

123

J. W. Squier
J. Stafford
H. H. Standen
E. Stangryciuk
(E. Black)
W. M. Stanley
H. Stannus
A. Stansberg
D. Stephen
D. W. R. Stewart
H. J. Stickings
P. Stoker
C. Stone
F. Strickland
G. A. Stroud
G. Struthers
D. Stults
J. B. Sullivan
A. K. Summerson
P. W. Sutton
F. Swain
L. Syrett
M. Szafranski
R. Tait
W. Tanner
R. Tarling
H. Taubman
B. Taylor
D. Taylor
E. A. Taylor
J. E. Taylor
G. F. Taylor
D. F. Tebbit
A. G. Thomas
J. Thomas
D. L. Thompson

J. J. Thompson
J. M. V. Thompson
G. W. Tiplady
A. H. Tollemache
J. J. Toper
J. Tosh
W. Towers-Perkins
K. N. Townsend
J. K. Trask
J. R. Treagust
L. Tremblay
F. Truhlar
K. S. Tugwell
L. Tully
R. Turnbull
G. Turner
J. Varty
J. Verran
D. L. Vince
E. Vincent
R. Vivian
T. E. Voges
L. Wainwright
A. E. Wakley
C. Walker
T. C. Walshe
K. C. Warburton
C. G. A. Ward
H. C. Ward
W. C. Warman
P. Warren
C. R. Warwick
J. T. Waterson
C. Watkins
F. Watkins
H. Watkins

P. J. Weber
F. Webster
P. C. Weeks
P. H. V. Wells
J. Welsh
J. Weston
F. V. Whale
B. G. Whalley
R. Wham
J. White
N. White
R. F. Whitehorn
M. W. E. Wild
C. Wilkes
L. R. Wilkins
G. Wilkinson
H. Williams
S. R. Williams
T. Williams
T. W. Williams
V. Willie
G. Wilson
M. Wilton
J. J. Wishart
I. A. Wood
H. W. Woodward
P. A. S. Woodwark
G. E. Wooley
A. Woolf
F. G. Woollard
R. Worn
D. Wright
C. M. Wright
J. E. F. Wright
R. C. Wright

*Note:* This list contains the names of all recorded Guinea Pigs.

# THE GUINEA PIG ANTHEM

We are McIndoe's army,
We are his Guinea Pigs.
With dermatomes and pedicles,
Glass eyes, false teeth and wigs.
And when we get our discharge
We'll shout with all our might:
'Per ardua ad astra,'
We'd rather drink than fight.

John Hunter runs the gas works,
Ross Tilley wields a knife.
And if they are not careful
They'll have your flaming life.
So, Guinea Pigs, stand steady
For all your surgeons' calls;
And if their hands aren't steady
They'll whip off both your ears.

We've had some mad Australians,
Some French, some Czechs, some Poles.
We've even had some Yankees,
God bless their precious souls.
While as for the Canadians –
Ah! That's a different thing.
They couldn't stand our accent
And built a separate Wing.

We are McIndoe's army,
(*As first verse.*)

# SCIENCE FICTION
## MONTHLY*

## A COLOURFUL NEW MAGAZINE-REVIEW

### Short stories, features, interviews and reviews covering the whole sphere of science-fiction.

First issue on sale January 31. Price 25p

Available at newsagents and bookstalls everywhere, or, if you should have any difficulty in obtaining your copy, available from the publishers, New English Library Ltd., price 30p (inclusive of postage and packing.)

---

### TO YOUR LOCAL NEWSAGENT

Please take note of my order for a regular monthly copy of 'SCIENCE-FICTION MONTHLY'.

Name .................................................................

Address .............................................................

...........................................................................

Price 25p monthly – First tremendous issue on sale January 31

**NEW ENGLISH LIBRARY LIMITED**
Barnard's Inn, Holborn, London EC1N 2JR. Tel: 01-405 4614.

---

*This magazine was previously announced as 'SCI-FI'. Any orders placed for 'SCI-FI' will, of course, stand for 'SCIENCE-FICTION MONTHLY'. The publishers apologise for any inconvenience caused by this change of title.

# NEL BESTSELLERS

| T011 682 | ESCAPE ON VENUS | *Edgar Rice Burroughs* | 40p |
|---|---|---|---|
| T013 537 | WIZARD OF VENUS | *Edgar Rice Burroughs* | 30p |
| T009 696 | GLORY ROAD | *Robert Heinlein* | 40p |
| T010 856 | THE DAY AFTER TOMORROW | *Robert Heinlein* | 30p |
| T016 900 | STRANGER IN A STRANGE LAND | *Robert Heinlein* | 75p |
| T011 844 | DUNE | *Frank Herbert* | 75p |
| T012 298 | DUNE MESSIAH | *Frank Herbert* | 40p |
| T015 211 | THE GREEN BRAIN | *Frank Herbert* | 30p |

## War

| T013 367 | DEVIL'S GUARD | *Robert Elford* | 50p |
|---|---|---|---|
| T013 324 | THE GOOD SHEPHERD | *C. S. Forester* | 35p |
| T011 755 | TRAWLERS GO TO WAR | *Lund & Ludlam* | 40p |
| T015 505 | THE LAST VOYAGE OF GRAF SPEE | *Michael Powell* | 30p |
| T015 661 | JACKALS OF THE REICH | *Ronald Seth* | 30p |
| T012 263 | FLEET WITHOUT A FRIEND | *John Vader* | 30p |

## Western

| T016 994 | No. 1 EDGE – THE LONER | *George G. Gilman* | 30p |
|---|---|---|---|
| T016 986 | No. 2 EDGE – TEN THOUSAND DOLLARS AMERICAN | | |
| | | *George G. Gilman* | 30p |
| T017 613 | No. 3 EDGE – APACHE DEATH | *George G. Gilman* | 30p |
| T017 001 | No. 4 EDGE – KILLER'S BREED | *George G. Gilman* | 30p |
| T016 536 | No. 5 EDGE – BLOOD ON SILVER | *George G. Gilman* | 30p |
| T017 621 | No. 6 EDGE – THE BLUE, THE GREY AND THE RED | | |
| | | *George G. Gilman* | 30p |
| T014 479 | No. 7 EDGE – CALIFORNIA KILLING | *George G. Gilman* | 30p |
| T015 254 | No. 8 EDGE – SEVEN OUT OF HELL | *George G. Gilman* | 30p |
| T015 475 | No. 9 EDGE – BLOODY SUMMER | *George G. Gilman* | 30p |
| T015 769 | No. 10 EDGE – VENGEANCE IS BLACK | *George G. Gilman* | 30p |

## General

| T011 763 | SEX MANNERS FOR MEN | *Robert Chartham* | 30p |
|---|---|---|---|
| W002 531 | SEX MANNERS FOR ADVANCED LOVERS | *Robert Chartham* | 25p |
| W002 835 | SEX AND THE OVER FORTIES | *Robert Chartham* | 30p |
| T010 732 | THE SENSUOUS COUPLE | *Dr. 'C'* | 25p |

## Mad

| S004 708 | VIVA MAD! | 30p |
|---|---|---|
| S004 676 | MAD'S DON MARTIN COMES ON STRONG | 30p |
| S004 816 | MAD'S DAVE BERG LOOKS AT SICK WORLD | 30p |
| S005 078 | MADVERTISING | 30p |
| S004 987 | MAD SNAPPY ANSWERS TO STUPID QUESTIONS | 30p |

---

NEL P.O. BOX 11, FALMOUTH, TR10 9EN, CORNWALL

Please send cheque or postal order. Allow 10p to cover postage and packing on one book plus 4p for each additional book.

Name ...........................................................................................................

Address...........................................................................................................

...........................................................................................................

Title ...........................................................................................................
(SEPTEMBER)